Fifty Minutes

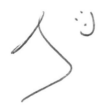

Fifty Minutes

Julie Webb

Matador
9 Priory Business Park,
Wistow Road, Kibworth Beauchamp,
Leicestershire. LE8 0RX
Tel: 0116 279 2299
Email: books@troubador.co.uk
Web: www.troubador.co.uk/matador
Twitter: @matadorbooks

ISBN 978 1838593 612

British Library Cataloguing in Publication Data.
A catalogue record for this book is available from the British Library.

Printed and bound in Great Britain by 4edge Limited
Typeset in 11pt Minion Pro by Troubador Publishing Ltd, Leicester, UK

Matador is an imprint of Troubador Publishing Ltd

Dad
1938-2020

Introduction

IT HAS BEEN ESTIMATED THAT THERE ARE OVER four hundred models of therapy, but I want to argue that there are as many models of therapy as there are therapists. However, all models pivot around a number of themes, some of which include acknowledging that the past influences the present; as bodies we experience powerful feelings that provide us with information; we form habits of thinking that influence our behaviour; relatedness is key to a sense of self; we live holding a constant tension that we will die. There is nothing medical in the themes listed here as they are all existential in nature.

The world of counselling and psychotherapy is constantly at odds with itself. That is a really good thing because in this sense the art of therapy in practice, resonates with what it is to exist as a human being: we are constantly at odds with ourselves. This being at odds seems to be a tension that we hold throughout our lives, not least because at a very early age we become aware of hurtling towards our own annihilation – death – realisation that can feel nonsensical, frightening, even cruel.

Whilst internally it may feel that we walk the earth alone holding this tension, we are also viscerally aware that we exist in a world full of others – people, animals, trees, mountains, fields and fauna. And not just others out there, but the sense of otherness within oneself. We could say that we are strangers to ourselves and that can create many tensions, for we want to be sure of ourselves, have a sense that we know who we are and feel strong and secure in our knowing. But what would it mean to *know thyself*, which is what many philosophical discourses, religious doctrines and therapeutic texts want to assert? And if I want to assert the opposite – that perhaps I do not know myself, that there is no self to know – who or what is it that is asserting? Well, there seems to be a body-mind consciousness in existence; a fleshy mass of hot blood that experiences thoughts and feelings, which seem to manifest and erupt from somewhere deep within and sometimes make the hair on my skin stand on end. It has an outward appearance of a form categorised as "woman" and functions as a woman – performs womanhood – an experiential performance that has been created by many influences such as biology, family, culture, society and psychology. It has been given the name Julie. The word Julie has become a signifier to refer to this fleshy mass sitting here. Though there are many Julies in the world, none are me.

If the "I" or "Julie" is just a signifier or referent point for this mass dwelling on earth, what am I articulating when I say there is no self to know? Well, what I want to say is that there is no fixed me and like a number of philosophers, poets and artists, I believe a firm identity is a poison and *know thyself* can be misleading. If I want to speak about myself I do so on the understanding that I may be quite unreliable, inconsistent, contradictory and paradoxical, and when I speak as a self I am probably referring to some set of beliefs I think I have in any given moment (including this one you understand). But the crucial point here is that a moment comes, and it goes, or rather the moment moves through me, and as it does so I cannot predict what it will bring with it and as such, I err towards those philosophical ideas that the "I" is an emergence – a primal, immanent vitality that is a constant beat. If you like, a constant moment-to-moment becoming. Poetic? I guess we have to be in the mood for poetics and when clients arrive for therapy feeling that life is not worth living, poetics is not what they want to hear, or often, are even able to hear. They want answers, a guide or manual, maybe an app with a set of instructions of how to get through their suffering or dilemma. Unfortunately, or I believe fortunately, there is no instruction manual and there are no answers. Really. As a therapist what I have is poetics: a lyrical curiosity to what appears in the therapeutic space; that I trust every person to have the capacity to work through their suffering; has the ability to weather storms; has the tenacity to dig deep and listen with their eyes and see with their ears to become attuned to the immanent vitality squirming deep down in the belly; that like all animals they instinctively know what they need and want. Needs and wants can often also be at odds with one another, particularly when experienced against a backdrop of capitalism, religion, social morality and family dynamics. But in fact, we need what we want and want what we need.

Therapy is one way of getting to the poetics of existence by engaging in the dance of person-to-person encounter, one-to-one or as part of a group, often in a small but comfortable room, sometimes during a walk in the park, occasionally via a computer screen or perhaps up a mountain and in the wild, wild woods. We will encounter words, silence, sometimes music, poetry, objects, movement. We are many different things and may require a diverse approach to aid a therapeutic journey.

Therapy can be an artistic activity to enquire and engage in the conflict felt within the body-mind system; tensions held between the referent "I" and the "other", both the stranger within and out there in the world; a path of reflection; a process to investigate dilemma. It is my belief that the best place counselling and psychotherapy can get to, is to aid a person to reach a point that when disturbance arises (and it will do so throughout the lifespan), she can be OK in it, even if she finds herself derailed. One might call this "resilience", which is the current buzzword in wellbeing parlance. The buzzword used to be "happy". Then we realised that we couldn't be happy all of the time. Maybe it's contentment – maybe that's the place we need to get to? Maybe. But I am interested in how we can be

OK in the discontentment of our ordinary daily lives. And how, if the discontentment is about social injustice, political reform or ethical encounter, can we fight and change things without becoming lost to despair or violent action? Therapy is like other art forms, it is political, social, personal, internal and external. How do these ideas play out in practice during therapy? Regardless of any sales pitch, therapists cannot know upfront what a client will bring, what the response will be, what will be felt, where the work will go. There is a trust that the journey will be where the client takes us and a faith that the therapist can not only be a companion on that unknown journey but can be open to being changed by it too. This notion places great emphasis on moment-to-moment experiencing and responsibility for how that experiencing is responded to. Often client work is to focus on the here and now, noticing and aiding a client to articulate what they are experiencing in the room when they are expressing something about their lives – whether past, present or future.

Not everyone sees therapy as an art form. It has become many things in our contemporary culture and the art form is currently under attack from bureaucrats; employers wanting us back to work speedily; producers wanting more production; medics wanting to cure; and clients wanting to be "fixed" because they have been sold the idea that therapy can "fix" people. People are not broken, even if they feel themselves to be. There is no cure for the human condition. None. A human being *is* neither a cancer nor a riddle. Though for sure, a human being can become ill and sometimes be confused and confusing.

And counselling and psychotherapy is not for capital gain, but for a sense of freedom and wellbeing for and in itself.

The collection of stories that follow offer descriptions of therapeutic encounter via fictional dialogues between client and therapist: snippets of someone's life fifty minutes at a time. They are ordinary stories about the ordinariness of life lived in a world with others. In reality the majority of work as a therapist is ordinary. Of course, we work with severe trauma, hideous abuse/violence, complex personality issues, terminal illness, but the majority of the work is working with human beings who are distressed, anxious, confused, or suffering a real sense of powerlessness and confusion in their everyday lives whilst they hold that constant tension of living/dying. That we all deal with the issues of the human condition is not to diminish anyone's suffering – some people clearly suffer and struggle more than others, in many different ways, and at different times throughout the lifespan.

Whatever a client is struggling with, language is going to be key. Language is powerful and not always clean; we muddy it, corrupt it and use it to manipulate – to remove honesty for all kinds of reasons – vulnerability, protection, gain and power. It is active, alive, always doing something, and no matter what kind of therapy we engage in – such as art therapy, dance, or writing – at some point we are going to talk about it. Words can hit the body both as friend and weapon. They can wake up the slumber of our complacent living with a short, sharp shock, and simultaneously confirm our lived experience, comforting enough to calm us to sleep. Language as a living phenomenon can craft our lives and our experience of the world, but it also gives us a platform from which to view the world. We all view the world through our own lens. If our view is that the world is a scary place then we are likely to live in accordance with that fear; if it is that God is the purveyor of all mankind then that is going to colour our view another way; if it is that there is a "them and us", then that will inform what choices we make and how we live out our life. And all of us – *all* – have a limited view of the world at any given moment and our view will be expressed within every encounter experienced. My current view derives from an understanding and unequivocal acceptance about our immanent nature and not fully knowing who or what we think we are, but what we *feel* ourselves becoming, and this necessarily raises questions about identity.

I have long been inquisitive about the subject of identity – what it is to want one, have one, lose one. And what it is to even speak of, as though it were a thing rather than a process. The question seems to perpetually produce itself when we feel a rupture, a sense of not belonging, not fitting, yearning and seeking. We all have identity even when attempting to escape such a notion. We have markers, categories, belongings. We seem to have a strong desire to belong to someone, something, and a hope that the belonging will somehow secure us and help us to become more stable and bigger than we actually are. We want to feel at home. And we are in fact homeless. We are all vagabonds masquerading as residents having arrived, because of course it is too disconcerting to feel lost at sea. So, we embellish our view, make comfort between the walls, shut our doors and turn the key in the lock.

The "I am" mode is precarious, deeply unstable and yet also creates a site for considerable striving, which sends a visceral insecurity through our blood that creates a constant and precious anxiety. Though acutely uncomfortable, this anxiety is our site of energy, freedom and creativity; A creative constant birthing which gives rise to the tension held within our finite existence and moment-to-moment decay. For if we are in a constant process of becoming, we are also in a constant process of undoing – shedding skins in order for the new to take its shape. In a way then, we are also in a constant state of grief.

Most of all, make no mistake that any sense we each have of "I" can only manifest and be experienced because there is "you". If I were lost to a desert island, I would have to find a football, draw a face on it and give it a name. That is how much I need all others. That we are inextricably bound to one another means that we truly, and without volition, are constantly gifted to one another. And of course, there is the downside when the gift is taken away. We are in a constant state of saying hello and goodbye both to ourselves in our moment-to-moment making, and to others who have been vital to that making. This is always both personal and political, whether we hold our personhood too tightly or force others to hold on to theirs.

Often it is painful to say goodbye or hear it said to us. We want to hold on, even if when we do, it does not serve us. Letting go is often a courageous endeavour and can create suffering somewhere and for someone. Loss seems to mean pain, anger, perhaps ailment and illness. Often it can make us feel that life is more precious than it really is and raise it to high grounds and pedestals. Equally it can make us fall to the doldrums, lash out and go under. But loss can be a gift because we cannot move forward, surge into, or rise above without it. How we hold the necessary tension of our experience in becoming/undoing and living/dying, can be a difficult and challenging task, often leaving a scar of some sort, somewhere. Loss creates a wound, but oh it is an honour to have cared so much to the point of being wounded so deeply.

Tess

'As I explained on the telephone, I don't have long left.' Her statement feels eager, hurried. A gentle, yet expectant smile eases its way through her face and flushes her cheeks as she takes a seat in the consulting room. I wait for her to settle before responding and notice an expectant flutter in my belly.

'I'm wondering what you would like to get from these sessions, Tess?'

'Well, I don't want to spend what little time I have left delving into my psyche! I just want to talk about me – my life, you know? I'm not looking for great changes or any change, I mean, nothing is going to change! I'm eighty-one and I am going to die – in a couple of months at the latest – this may be the only session – you probably want to do more.'

'You can talk about whatever you want for just one session if that's what you need.'

'I've had a nice life, well more than nice really.' She brushes her skirt as though there were fluff on it. '*Nice* is such an empty word, isn't it? Meaningless.'

'It's hard to find the right word sometimes I think, but I hear "nice" isn't the right one for you.'

'No. I've had a really lovely life, lovely. Nothing spectacular, quite ordinary really and I had a lovely husband with whom I shared fifty-five years, three children and seven grandchildren. I was a teacher too – I told you that on the phone, sorry if I'm repeating myself.'

'Sounds like your life has been full.'

'Yes, it has been, is, but I don't want to talk about my family particularly or work even – I retired a long time ago. I think I've sacrificed enough of myself for them.'

'It's been a sacrifice.'

'Of course! To be married that long to bring up stable children and help with grandchildren, you have to put yourself on hold sometimes to do that well.'

'Being on hold was necessary and important for you.'

'Yes, it was a priority once I'd decided to surrender to that kind of life.'

'You surrendered consciously to a particular kind of life.'

'Yes. It's a huge commitment to stay married, all the ups and downs and focus on the children you have chosen to bring into the world.'

'An important commitment for you.'

'I haven't always got it right, done it well, but I think I can say I tried my damnedest.' She pauses slightly, then looks me dead in the eye. 'I'm out-of-date now, old fashioned.'

We sit for a few moments as Tess surveys the room. I feel a little uneasy, not sure why. She is articulate; her tone of voice is both gentle and confident, formidable. She was a schoolteacher and taught English. I notice I feel warm towards her and remember as a child my own dream of becoming a teacher, though I'd always imagined myself to be rather like Margaret Rutherford, all buxom and tweedy. Tess is more Charlotte Rampling – slim, soft, rosy-cheeked with warm eyes. I expected her eyes to be cold and dark as they are dying but no, they seem full of spring somehow. She is smart, classic. Dressed in a black, long slim skirt; white, crisp cotton blouse, mustard-coloured long cardigan, and shiny black patent shoes that form a mirror to the body standing in them.

'I had a dream the other night, which is what prompted me to call you. Well two dreams actually, back-to-back the same night. In the first one I woke myself up screaming, got up, made a cup of tea and went back to sleep and had the second dream. But it was strange, like they were connected.'

'Sounds powerful, two connecting dreams.'

'Yes, I think they were my body talking and preparing me.'

'Your body talks to you through your dreams.'

'Of course.'

She knows more about this business than me it seems.

'I was sat in a café and had finished my coffee. I paid the waitress, picked up my bag – not this one,' touching the shiny black patent one at her feet, another mirror matching her shoes, 'another one I have with flowers on it, though in the dream the flowers were too bright, artificial like in a Disney film if you know what I mean? I knew in the dream I recognised the bag, it was mine and it felt very real. I was going to meet someone but I couldn't grasp who. It felt OK though. As I walked out of the café I was in a kind of department store and had to take a lift to get out of the building to meet the person I was going to meet. So I got in the lift with other people. When the doors opened for my floor I got out. I was the only one. Then as I looked around I noticed the whole floor of the store had been concreted over: walls, windows, ceiling, everything grey, smooth concrete. I felt panicked and turned to get back in the lift only to see the doors close shut and disappear as the wall sealed itself in concrete. In that moment I had a vile feeling that ran through me, like black freezing water filling my veins and felt that if I screamed no one would hear me. I was entombed and going to die and no one knew I was there. That's when I woke myself up screaming. I can feel my heart racing just talking about it. I felt death. I'm sure of it.'

'It's a dramatic description of being sealed in what appears like a concrete tomb.'

'Well… in a way it makes sense that I'm frightened of dying without anyone knowing.' Her eyes fill with tears. 'Nobody wants to die alone do they, even if we all do… really… in the end?' We sit quietly for a moment or two and I notice my own sadness gently rise. 'I felt sheer fear when I realised I was going to die in there. I didn't feel that sensation when the doctors first told me, but I did in the dream, suddenly breathless.'

'In the dream you had a visceral realisation that you were going to die and it took your breath away.'

'Yes.'

I watch this woman alive, thinking and talking, and for all the world looking radiant. She had contained herself in her attire for the day ahead to discuss her memories and feelings about her life with me and she is dying before my eyes. I don't know her and I don't want her to die. How stupid the thought, the feeling, that my body just produced – my wants like they have any reality to them.

'It frightened me and I guess that's why I woke myself up screaming.'

'You say "woke yourself up", like there was some intent.'

'Yes, I think there was, don't you? That my body couldn't cope with the fear it was feeling so it woke me up for safety.'

'Waking up kept you safe.'

'I think maybe I could've died in the dream otherwise.'

'You felt the dream brought you closer to death.'

'In a way, but it's like I said, "Nope – not like this, and not now".'

'You chose.'

'Hmm… maybe. The dream that followed is what settled me to think that.'

'In what way?'

'Well it was almost a repeat of the first dream being in the café. Only this time after I paid the waitress and made my way to the lift, I knew I was meeting my husband. And I did, just in the foyer by the lift he was waiting for me. We got into the lift holding hands. Then as the doors began to close I woke up naturally.'

'The difference between the two dreams is that in the second you knew that you were with your husband getting into the lift. You didn't get out of the lift?'

'No.'

'What feelings, if any, do you remember about that second dream?'

'Oh they were lovely feelings, warm, loving, soft and gentle. I thought "ahh, he has come to collect me" and I felt very, very safe, a lot different to the first dream.'

'Love, gentle, safe. No fear this time.'

'No. But I'm confused, because actually I could've gone then.'

'What do you mean "gone"?'

'I could've gone with him, died in my sleep with him holding my hand. Isn't that what we would read in stories? Nice and neat, me heading towards the light with my dead husband holding my hand guiding me over.'

'Sounds like a cliché?'

'Yes! Exactly that. Though it was comforting I have to say.'

'The cliché is a comfort.'

'Yes. I don't want to die with the feeling of the first dream.'

'Yes, I can appreciate that and I can also appreciate how fearful it can be to not know how we will feel when the moment comes.'

'It's not so much that.'

'Oh.' We sit for another moment or two silently. She presses her lips together and then opens them slightly as her tongue swirls around in her mouth.

'When I was thirty-two I had an affair. I think now that he was the love of my life.' She seems to rest herself in the statement as her eyes glance at me, then swiftly disconnect in the exposure.

'The "love of your life" is a powerful declaration.'

'Yes, it is, isn't it? And true. We'd meet in his flat. He lived above the Chinese takeaway. We'd eat chicken chow mein in the afternoons – disgustingly chewing on food with our mouths wide open to share the mastication. Then we'd spit it into each other's mouths. It was exquisite. We'd just talk and eat and love each other. It was so simple. It had to end of course. I had two children by then and a husband – responsibilities. He was a couple of years younger than me doing his PhD.'

'Responsibilities forced an ending.'

'No, it wasn't that. I knew the spitting and loving wouldn't last, it couldn't, you see. That kind of meeting, that kind of intensity, cannot last.'

'The intensity was unsustainable.'

'Yes. Although we had three glorious years. But it was more than that, I was determined not be *that* person who left. And I had promised – and was also too cowardly – to experience the pain I could feel bubbling in me or watch the pain that I knew would be inflicted upon the family. Though when I ended the affair I thought I would die from the pain it was so intense.' She looks up at me and smiles. 'Of course, I didn't.'

'You made promises and also felt too cowardly to experience the pain.'

'Yes, a bit like the fear in the dream when I thought I was going to die.'

'You were frightened.'

'Yes, but the intensity was awful anyway, so really no matter what I did I was going to suffer but it wasn't all about me, you see.'

'Yes, I see that.' Quiet surrounds us but is broken by the traffic coming from outside. The reality of our existence outside of these four walls is a noisy one.

'You see, what I didn't say was that although I felt safe after my second dream, I also felt disappointed.'

'Disappointed how?'

'That it wasn't my lover holding my hand as I got into the lift.' She sits a little upright and wriggles in her seat, reaching for the glass of water on the table to her side, though I am certain she is not thirsty. She glances back with her eyes full of spring and holds the glass in front of her face as though it were a prism to produce a Picasso work of art.

'You wanted it to be your lover holding your hand.'

'I know it's selfish. I had given so much, I just wanted one last glance.'

'A last glance.'

'Yes.' She cradles the glass of water as tears stream down her face. 'Stupid isn't it, the hopes we hold on to?'

'It feels stupid.'

'Yes, I feel stupid. I feel like I'm thirty-two again. I don't think those feelings ever left me.'

'Like they're frozen in time.'

'Exactly like that. But then that's why I ended it, isn't it? To freeze it so that it didn't decay. I wish I hadn't in so many ways. And yet also glad I did. I don't know what I'm talking about, I feel like I'm babbling.'

'It sounds like you are a woman coming to the end of her life and wondering what life may've been like if she'd made different choices. I hear that you're happy with the choices and decisions that you made but also deeply sad with grief at what you also gave up. I also hear how you would like just one last glance, one moment to feel those feelings with your lover one last time.'

Tess sits and cries with sobs breaking free. It takes some time for them to subside as her body settles into composure.

'There I've said it all,' she says through a deep sigh.

'You feel it's all said.'

'Yes. I just wanted to say it to someone before I died. Before… before I go and meet my husband at the lift.' She grins playfully and I find myself grinning with her.

'You wanted to share your feelings.'

'Yes. It's simple really, isn't it. Can I tell you one more thing?'

'Of course, go ahead.'

'When my husband died, three years ago, I wasn't there. He had a heart attack in his shed. I was napping. When I started to come around from sleep – you know that strange state between sleep and awake feeling?' I nod. 'Well, I realised I was cold, but almost immediately this sensation of warm water flooded my body from the top of my head to my feet. Then I felt the weight of the blanket on me, which was strange, I thought, because it was just a light shawl really, and I somehow immediately knew that there was a person lying next to me on top of the blanket causing it to be pulled tight. I reached out my hand and as I turned, it was my husband. I knew in an instant he'd died, and I heard his voice say, "It's alright." Then I woke up properly, sat up and looked through the window into the garden. I felt stupidly calm as I walked through the house and into the garden towards the shed, I knew he'd gone, I knew. Of course it was horrible. My best friend had gone.'

'What a powerful scene and I notice even though you are describing the death of your husband and best friend, that I feel warm.'

'Yes, strange, isn't it, I felt warm too. He always made me feel warm. Even in his last moment, he came to comfort me.' She stares and smiles. I'm just about holding my tears in a well at the back of my throat.

Tess looks at the clock and I look at the clock. 'Thank you for your time today,' she says through a smile. 'I don't think I'll come again though. I think I will be alright now.'

A thud of disappointment drops hard to the bottom of my body. I want to talk with her more; stupid, but I really don't want her to leave, or die.

'If you feel at any point you'd like to talk again then do please get in touch, Tess – anytime. It was good to meet you today.'

'Thank you.'

Meg

'TODAY WOULD BE MY MOTHER'S BIRTHDAY. SHE killed herself five years ago – she was seventy-three. She left a letter, said she wanted some peace. I could never convince her that she needed to be alive to know peace; I mean when you're dead, you're dead.'

I say nothing and cannot detect any emotion in these statements.

'She did say that she was sorry she had to go now but that everyone has their time and this could be the only time that she could "win at life". Suddenly a smirk saunters across her face. 'She said she loved me, and all that usual stuff, but I've always been sceptical as I don't feel that she really had any capacity to love anyone except my father, who she was with for five minutes and ran off the minute he heard about me. I don't know what my mother meant by love.' We sit for a few moments as she sighs heavily, almost *tuts*.

'That was a big sigh, Meg.'

'When love goes wrong, I feel I've somehow got life wrong.'

'Life feels wrong when love goes wrong, Meg?'

'Yes.' Her eyes fill and she shuffles in her seat. Moving her body to delay the stream somehow.

'I have refused all my life to live like she did.'

'You insist on living differently.'

'There were suicide attempts when I was little, constant grieving for the phantom twat of a man. She was depressed most of the time, isolated and lost in bloody Judy Garland films – you know *The Man that Got Away*? I know she pined but years and bloody years of it.'

'She was stuck? And you sound irritated. How little were you when she attempted suicide?'

'Seven. I remember walking into the sitting room and there she was crawling around on her knees, mumbling and putting her fingers into the electric sockets, flicking the switches on and off – can you die from that? I think I might've laughed, but ran out to fetch my aunt Pam, Mum's sister. Mum went into hospital for two weeks though it felt much longer than that. I didn't see her until she came home again. She acted as though nothing had happened, and yet somehow, I knew that she, and everything in life from then on, was completely changed. All she ever said, which was more a slip of the tongue years later, was that "they fried my brain".'

'Walking in on that scene changed life forever.'

'Yes, but… I don't really want to talk about her. I've done therapy before and done enough work on that area of my life.'

'You've talked enough about that.'

'Yes, done that story to death.'

We sit in a pause, waiting for the next words to emerge.

'I mean it was irritating. She wouldn't… she just point-blank refused to get on with life.'

'She was stuck.'

'You said that earlier.'

'I did. And I'm aware that you said you didn't want to talk about her anymore and yet here you are, stuck with that story.'

'You think I'm stuck?'

'I'm curious that you find yourself talking about something that you say you don't want to.'

'From what I can remember, she had few relationships. But she'd be devastated every time one ended.' Meg raises her arms. 'I mean ab-so-lute-ly devastated. She'd curl up in foetal position, like a child with a teddy on the bed, holding *the* photograph of my father. Judy Garland's *The Man that Got Away* would be turning on the record player repeatedly. I fucking hate that song – I mean women have moved on from that, haven't they?'

'What was it like for you to watch her devastation?' Her stare pierced through me. I feel the words "her devastation" jarred somehow.

'I hated it. I've never known my father. The story goes that he disappeared when he got wind of my impending birth. I'm pretty sure that I felt my mother's shock as I came out two months too early. Mum was only eighteen when she had me.' We sit for what seems an age and I feel my eagerness to want to know what she's pondering on as she sits there staring at the floor. 'I've never been interested in wanting to know anything about him, she was enough, in all sorts of ways. I got the gist that they dated for a couple of months and that he was always restless and filled her head with lots of plans to travel. I can only imagine the panic he must've felt… anyhow… shitty thing to do though, just fucking off without a word. Mum carried a photo of him everywhere she went. I considered *the* photo to be the cause of most of her suffering. I buried it with her as requested, though I wanted to burn the fucking thing.'

I notice that the "f" in "fucking" sounds like it is ten-feet-tall and in bold type.

'You sound angry.'

'I am. I mean what a fucking waste of a life.'

'Whose?'

'Well, hers, of course.'

'You feel she wasted her life.'

'Yes, of course she did. She did nothing but wallow. She was bright, funny, pretty, articulate. She could've lived.'

'You don't feel that she lived.'

'Not any kind of life that I consider living.'

'What is a living kind of life for you, Meg?'

'Well not moping around in bed crying over a fleeting lover.'

'From your description, it sounds like your father felt to be more than a fleeting lover to your mother.' Meg looks cross and diverts her eyes away from me. 'You didn't like what I said.'

'No. Well. It doesn't matter really. You're right, it all felt much more to her.'

'But it angered you when I offered that?'

'Yes, well mostly, I dunno.'

Meg sits for a few minutes. I have this feeling that although she seems angry or irritated about her mother's depression, whatever is going on is not about her mother.

'D'you think we ever get over stuff, you know, *really* get over stuff?'

'What would really getting over stuff be for you, Meg?'

'That I wouldn't still be thinking about it – the pain nearly killed me when she died and I felt like I'd run out of time too.' Her eyes glisten with salt. 'And it's happened again, though no one has died.' She brushes a stray curl from her face and turns her head to the wall as she speaks to me. 'My lover has ended our relationship.' Pained eyes stare back at me. 'Just like that.'

'Loss brings a feeling of running out of time for you. You speak as though this recent ending caught you by surprise.'

'I must've seen it coming yet I feel so shocked. We were pretty stable, I thought, you know, we had a good understanding after all these years – twenty, twenty years. I loved him – love him – very much. And I didn't surrender lightly all those years ago – he pursued me. I have to be in awe of a man if there is any chance of me falling in love with him. Even in awe of his stupidity and arrogance, for we are all that, eh.' She giggles, slightly throwing her head back, masking any pain she might be feeling and I'm aware that I'm searching her face for pain.

'This was a significant relationship and you felt shocked when it ended.'

'Yes.' Her eyes fill. 'I feel bereft.' She can barely form her words through the contorted mouth. 'I keep replaying events over and over in my head and I don't understand what's changed. We've been seeing each other twenty years – twenty years!' She repeats and holds her hands out, palms skyward. 'It's a long time, you know.'

'It is.' I nod.

'Twenty years of my life.'

'You've given twenty years of your life to the relationship and don't understand what changed for it to end like this.'

'Yes. I gave.' Tears stream down her face. 'Now what? I'm sixty years old, now what?' Meg sits and sobs. I leave her to her tears, keeping eye contact should she need company.

'We made love with words… his mouth carried meaning for me as though he knew all my world with his words. Sometimes, I would have to kiss his lips when he was speaking. Like an attempt to eat his words. It felt as though if I could just eat and be full, then the yearning would cease. I wanted to rest there forever on his mouth. So stupid, stupid.' She shakes her head ferociously and I think of Tess and her insistence that intensity cannot last and I notice that I don't want to believe that is the case.

'You feel stupid for wanting to rest forever on his mouth and feel full. It sounds intense, poetic.'

'It was… or that's what I thought it was… it's so pathetic I know, and I know I should know better. But I love him so much and even though we rarely saw each other I felt it to be real, meaningful, worthy. For both of us – not just me – it wasn't just me! I feel like some stupid schoolgirl who should've known better.'

'You feel young, naive, stupid.'

She can't speak now through her tears and just cries. I notice the immaculate ruby red paint on her toes poking through her sandals, which are like walking sandals, old and tatty. Whilst the toes are still, they look defiant and insistent upon demanding to be noticed in the contrast. The rest of her is dressed in white, which sets off jet wisps on the underside of her pinned grey hair. She looks at me with her intense blue, somewhat Celtic eyes, wipes her face and blows her nose.

'I've written countless messages and poems to him but not sent them. I want to write an old-fashioned letter and drip a tear onto the page, tear it out and send it in an envelope, you know, with SWALK on the seal. Maybe I should email it, text it? Let him know. But… what if he doesn't understand my love? I felt so sure, now everything is… lost, uncertain, gone.' She folds her arms across her body as if holding herself.

'You want to make him see how painful this is for you and how your body feels lost and uncertain. Something feels gone and I notice how you hold your body as if to make sure it is there.'

'Yes, I feel lost in my body. I feel unreal somehow – what am I now?'

'You've lost a sense of yourself.'

'Yes. What am I without him in my life?' She stares at the picture on the wall, or rather through the picture, and I feel a conflict within me. Do I sit and wait out her next move or do I offer an observation? A tussle going on inside me.

'Meg, I recall near the beginning of our session when you were talking about your mum, that you said when love goes wrong, it feels like "you've" got life wrong somehow. I noticed you weren't referring to your mother in that statement. I'm wondering if your sense of getting life wrong has any bearing upon your loss somehow?' She looks startled. *Fuck.* I wonder what she heard in my question. I wait a really long time…

'He was married.'

'I see.'

'You think I've no right to grieve?' She is stony-faced staring at me, daring me.

'I don't think grief is about rights. You had a twenty-year, deeply significant relationship and your grief is real, palpable, I see you're suffering.'

'But everyone said "he's unavailable, Meg", they told me.'

'Unavailable.'

'Unavailable. Time-limited. That's not what they meant, they meant it couldn't go anywhere. But I was really OK where we were. I'd never wanted him to leave her. It would've killed a vital part in him. And I never wanted the claustrophobia of marriage and clearly neither did he otherwise he wouldn't have been seeing me!'

'He was unavailable in a time-limited sense and the relationship really worked for you.'

'Yes.'

I notice I feel a doubt.

'Well, no, not just time, I mean because there was little time he wasn't really there for me emotionally – he couldn't – sometimes when I needed him to be.'

'Emotional support was lacking at times.'

'Well yes, but because there was no time.'

'Time was the reason.' We sit in silence for a moment or two.

'Men are such fuckers, aren't they?'

'Men are?'

'Yes, they swan around coming and going as they please. You know, when I got divorced nothing changed for my husband, other than I wasn't there. He just carried on with his career, got himself another woman really quick and married again – *bam* – just like that.'

'Men can just do things *bam* just like that – your lover ended your relationship just like that and your ex-husband got on with life just like that and your father left just like that.'

'Yeah, does anything really touch them? Does it?'

'In the way that things touch you.' She breaks down again.

'I loved my husband very much but I couldn't stay, I couldn't thrive and I felt stifled and stuck.'

'You had to leave your marriage because you felt stifled and stuck.'

'Silly really, in the end.'

'Why silly?'

'Because in a way my feeling that way wasn't anything to do with the marriage, it was to do with something deep in me. I mean I've done a lot of work on myself to come to that conclusion – all a bit late I know.'

'Late, in what way?'

'Well, I just think if I'd known then what I know now we could've worked through it all.'

'You have regrets.'

'Sometimes, no, yes… not really, it was all the right thing to do at the time. Whatever was wrong or whatever it was I needed wasn't met by Richard – that's my ex-husband. But Len, everything was met, it was all there.'

'Your needs weren't met by Richard in your marriage but unavailable Len met all your needs.'

'Oh, that was clever.'

'How so?'

'Unavailable Len met all my needs you said. Sounds sarcastic – like, how could he meet all my needs if he was unavailable is what you're really asking.'

'Am I?'

'Of course he didn't meet all my needs but he met those really important needs in me.'

'Needs that are important to you were met by Len.'

'Yes – he was attentive, he understood, you know – he just got it – we shared poetry, music, we read to each other – there was this – this mutual understanding – yes like a mutual meeting. We just got each other. I felt seen, known.'

'You felt met, seen and known with shared mutual interests and understanding.'

'Y-e-s.' She nods through tears as the broken word leaves her mouth. I notice our time running out but she is quite distressed.

'Sounds very powerful and important to you to feel met, seen and known, Meg.'

Through nods and broken words, 'Yeah, it feels so hard… so lonely, which is stupid 'cause I was always alone but as long as he was in the world and we were connected I felt whole, I did… and now…' She suddenly changes, sits upright, waves her arms in the air and her face becomes taut. 'Now, I sound like my bloody mother.'

'You sound angry.'

'I don't want to get swallowed by this pain like she did. I don't want it, I don't.'

We sit for a moment as that statement rests and her tears subside, allowing the end of the session to feel more natural.

Luke

FROM THE BEGINNING LUKE'S EXISTENCE FELT LIKE a growing boil. In his youth he was always throbbing and hot, except in the middle of the night when he woke freezing and his joints ached from being curled up into the tightest ball. During the school day his face would burn with shame most of the time. It is shameful to never quite measure up. The inside of his belly would feel swollen, tender and sore, his head muddled and confused, and his eyes sometimes could not see straight. Through panic he would momentarily go deaf, and the world became a frightening muffle. And then one day via an almighty grief in middleage, the boil burst and, slowly, a raw, courageous freeself began to grow in its place.

I greet Luke in reception as I have done so for eighteen months now. I hover in the doorway smiling and he looks up, phone in hand to look like he has something to do rather than just being able to sit still in a silent space with strangers. It is the modern way.

As I sit down, I watch him put his keys and phone on the table beside his seat and then drop down, lead-like into it. Air expels from his body as he looks at me with expectant eyes. He wants something. He reaches for the glass of water and takes a sip. I don't think he really wants to sip his water but it is something to do in the silence, waiting for something to start, not realising it has already begun. We settle into our seats and sit in silence for a while. Luke breaks it.

'How are you?'

'I'm well, thank you. How are things with you, Luke?' This is a choice point. I could've equally not asked how he is and made him squirm a little longer in the silence. Sometimes we all need a little invitation.

'Yeah, OK, alright. Haven't slept much this week.'

'Yes, you look a little tired around your eyes and I noticed the big sigh as you seemed to collapse into your seat.'

'I'm tired; been difficult to concentrate on work this week.' I hear traffic and emergency sirens en route to the hospital down the road. 'I like the peace in here, probably why I fell into the chair – relief.' He half-heartedly smiles.

'Feels like a relief falling into the chair in this peaceful setting.'

'Yeah.'

I hear my stomach rumble loudly, like it is amused and I smile, placing my hands on my belly.

'You sound hungry,' he said.

'I am a little.'

'No breakfast?'

'Not enough.'

'I haven't had breakfast all week,' he said, 'ran out of time every morning. I just couldn't get out of bed when the alarm went off. It's driving Cherry and the kids mad, especially at the weekend.'

'You're having difficulty getting out of bed, Luke?'

'Yeah. My body just feels so heavy. It's like I just can't pick it up.'

'You speak as though your body is not part of you and it is too heavy to lift.'

'It doesn't feel part of me. It feels like a big heavy lump that I'm dragging around.'

'There is you,' I raise my left hand, 'and then this big heavy lump,' I raise my right hand, 'you are having to drag around with you,' and I bring my hands together, his eyes following the motion. 'Sounds like a real effort, Luke.'

'It is, it really is.' The heavy silence fills up the space between us and I can feel my energy beginning to drop into the seat. Things had been going well for Luke lately and his energy was on the rise. Today feels low.

'I notice I feel my own energy drop, something in the air feels heavy, Luke; weighty somehow, I don't know – the word "looming" is coming up for me.'

'Yeah, yeah that's it, it's just all looming.' His eyes connect with mine as if to give further endorsement that the word found is the right one. He sits up ever so slightly as his shoulders eek a millimetre forward.

'Something's looming.'

'Yeah, and it's heavy, pushing me down.' His shoulders drop.

'Whatever "it" is, is looming heavy above you and is pushing you down. I notice your shoulders drop.'

His eyes start to fill and his cheeks become red. He looks away to the window with his mouth quivering. I wait a while as redness and tears shape the air. I feel my own face come to stillness and keep my eyes focused on the client as I watch him work hard to control the emotion.

'You look like you're trying really hard not to cry. I see your eyes filled and your mouth quivering.'

'It's just, it's too…' Words get stuck as tears silently roll down. He stifles a sob and grabs a tissue from the box. I think about some of the crass anecdotes about therapists having tissues on the table, making crying an expectation in therapy. Well I want to say, we also have heating on in the room, a chair to sit on, light and preferably a window. I also put a jug of water out and a glass in case client or therapist gets thirsty. It seems to me, given the nature of the work, that tissues may also be of help, a basic need you might say when tears and snot are streaming from one's face. Who the devil am I imagining saying this to? Luke blows his nose, which somehow stops the tears.

'It just feels too hard.'

'Something feels too hard, Luke.'

'Rebecca wants me to leave Cherry and the kids, and I, I just… I can't, it's just too hard, I can't even think about it… it churns me up inside.'

'Thinking about leaving churns you up.'

'Yeah, like right here, I feel sick.' He scrunches his gut. 'Look how much weight I've put back on. I haven't been to the gym in weeks.'

'How come, what's changed for you?'

'Seeing Rebecca more. I say I'm going to the gym but I'm seeing her. Last night Cherry said, "That gym doesn't seem to be paying off".'

'What did it feel like when she said that?'

'I felt guilty and panicked. I'll have to start going again or else she'll suspect. Well, I think she does anyway. She reckoned you're not much cop because I seem to be going backwards.'

'What d'you think she meant by backwards?'

'That my weight is coming back, that I'm tired all the time, not sleeping. I snapped at the kids the other night.'

'You're snappy and tired and that feels like a backward step.'

'According to her, yeah. But in a way, I feel I've moved such a long way. When I'm with Rebecca I feel so alive and she doesn't care if I'm carrying weight and not going to the gym.'

'You feel alive with Rebecca. What is it when you are with her that makes you feel alive?'

'Well she just gets me. I don't have to really do anything; she's very self-sufficient. Her place is peaceful and tidy, no kids' stuff everywhere. I like the quiet, though we talk a lot about stuff. Cherry's not that into talking much, and she doesn't like sport, whereas Rebecca really loves sport and we wanna just go to matches and stuff but can't really be seen out, you know. It's all cloak and dagger.' He smiles, almost chuckles as he lowers the volume and yet deepens his voice when he says "cloak and dagger".

'Sounds like Rebecca meets an important part of you that likes sport and a peaceful, uncluttered setting where you don't have to do anything. I noticed your energy rise when you said "cloak and dagger" and you sounded playful, cheeky. You chuckled slightly but lowered your voice.'

'Yeah, it feels naughty, a secret and that makes it lighter. Home is heavy.'

'Home feels heavy for you and your secret makes life naughty and light.'

'It's not Cherry's fault. She is busy, you know, with the kids, and her mum is ill, and so she is trying to look after her and keep an eye on her dad as well. She works really hard to keep everyone happy. I feel I let her down.'

'I notice when I said "life feels lighter and naughty" you immediately gave me a rundown of how busy Cherry is caring for everyone and that you feel you let her down.'

'She does, and here I am being a shit and cheating on her. A year ago, I'd never have done this.' He pronounces each word fully.

'You feel like a shit. What do you attribute to your change of behaviour this last year?'

'Well all the work we've done and lancin' that boil that seemed to dog me all my life. I felt I could do anything, was more confident and that gave me more energy and a sense of purpose. I liked myself. But I lost it again and now it's all murky again. I worry I might go back to that place and I don't want to.'

'Sounds like a bit of a rollercoaster. You lanced the boil, felt great, had purpose and liked yourself and now it's got all murky again.'

'Yeah. Exactly. I was down, then up flying high, now I'm down and don't want to go to the bottom 'cause it's hard getting back up on top.'

We sit in silence for a moment or two, Luke with his head down and my gaze firmly upon him. He lifts his head and in a small, tender voice says, 'I was thinking, I dunno if I want to be at the top again. I mean it felt good, but it changed things.'

'Things changed when you were at the top of the ride?'

He responds with a light self-mocking chuckle, 'Yeah, maybe I got a bit cocky and thought I could fly.'

'The high costs you somehow?'

'Yeah, that's exactly it; it felt great, but didn't pay off the way I'd have liked – well it did and didn't all at the same time.'

'So, you seem to be saying there is a tension that you are having to hold between the pay-off and the cost: it paid off and didn't all at the same time.' I gesture as though holding the opposite ends of taut rope.

He nods with his head down, looking at his own hands.

'You know what you said a few weeks ago about there's no straight line, I get it now. It was hard getting to feeling better about things, all that stuff as a kid in school and my anxiety. I thought when I got there, felt better, that'd be it, sorted. But it's not, is it? Is it ever sorted? I really can't face going down to the bottom again.'

'I don't hold the belief that there is a straight line through the process no, but what I really hear is how much you can't face being at the bottom again. Mmm… I'm wondering what might be different for you this time, Luke, if anything?'

'What d'you mean?'

'Well, you're not at the bottom yet. When you first came here you were at the bottom, almost beyond the bottom.'

'Yeah, I was, wasn't I?'

'Do you have options or choices that if you reached the bottom, it might be different to being at the bottom from last time?'

'Oh, I see. I suppose I know what that feels like so I can do something about it earlier maybe? I'm coming here, whereas I wasn't last time until it was nearly too late. Cherry now knows about a lot of this stuff I hadn't told her before.'

'How might any of that help you at all?'

'It's different I suppose and seeing that I was able to get up out of that hole means I can again, I guess.'

'And you're not in the hole yet.'

'True.'

'If you did fall back into the hole, is there any part of the experience that might be a pay-off. By that I mean, might you gain something?'

'Oh fuck, I ain't ever going back into that. I'd lose Cherry and the kids for good. I'd lose everything. I don't even want to think about it. I can't. I can't go there… I can't…' He shakes his head profusely and his eyes dart around the room.

'The cost would be too high and you sound panicky, Luke.'

'This is the feeling I get in the middle of the night. It just swirls around and around.' He shuffles in his seat.

'The thoughts of losing Cherry and the kids, losing everything, swirl around and around and keep you awake and panicky.'

He breaks again and tears roll, as his body twitches and glances at the closed door. He has bolted before and we have both worked hard to help him stay with the panic and remain in the room.

'You look panicked and jumpy, Luke.'

'I can't stand the feeling, I can't lose her, I can't...'

'Breathe, Luke, the panic is just a feeling.' I mouth a slow breath for him to mimic. 'Take a breath... slow... breathe... get the oxygen into your body... remember what we've done before, locate the feeling and stay with it... lean into it with your breath... stand if you need to... move the energy... and breathe... I can really hear your panic, so breathe with the feeling and hold its hand. Remember your breathing... slow... slow.'

He shifts in his seat and an almighty sob escapes and takes him by surprise. He darts a look at me. It takes a while for Luke to really slow his breathing, and tears become silent as they leave his eyes more freely. He grabs more tissues and blows a handful of snot out of his system. We just sit and I feel myself relax as the air around us begins to still. I wait a few moments more for his breathing to become normal and his tears to subside.

'We just have a minute or two left, Luke. I just want to check you're alright to go back out into the day.'

'Yeah, yeah I'm OK. I'm OK. I didn't expect that. It came up from my boots.'

'Yes, it looked like it had been waiting. We are booked in for the same time next week, is that still alright, Luke?'

'Yeah. OK. Thanks.' He stands, throws a handful of tissues in the bin. 'Can I?' He gestures towards a bowl of sweets that I keep on the table.

'Of course, go ahead.' I long for the day that he just takes the sweet without asking. Though my longing will cease the moment he leaves the room. I stand too and head towards the door, giving him one last glance before I turn the door handle, 'OK?'

'Yep.'

As I open the door a wave of cool air wafts in as Luke walks out.

Rosie

ROSIE AND I SIT OPPOSITE EACH OTHER, SMILING.

'I don't know what to say,' she opens.

'Yes, it can be hard to know where to start. Maybe you could say something about what brings you here, why now?'

'My friend suggested it really... I mean I wanted to come, I've been really tearful lately and... oh...' she bursts into sobs and grabs a handful of tissues from the box. I feel myself sit up a little straighter. 'Sorry, I didn't expect that, I've been fine, really.'

'The tears have taken you by surprise.'

'Yeah, a bit, but as I said I've been tearful but I've coped quite well, I didn't expect to feel like this.'

'You've been coping well and your feelings have bubbled up unexpectedly.' Rosie nods as she blows a head full of snot into the tissue. I can see she is finding it hard to hold back her tears and she is insistent upon composing herself.

As she begins to speak, she breaks down again, stops herself suddenly with wide eyes peering at me over the handful of tissues held to her face, 'I'm sorry, I don't know where it's coming from.' She shakes her head at me as she speaks.

'Well it looks like it wants to come up, maybe we should just let it.' And she does, for what seems like ages. I notice the tissue box emptying and swiftly produce another one.

'I'm sorry, I've used all your tissues.'

We sit in the quiet for a few moments after Rosie has stopped crying. She tosses all the used wet tissues resting on her lap into the bin and takes a new, crisp, clean one and folds it in between her fingers.

'Hoh. That was a lot. I didn't realise all that was there.'

I just smile at her and give her the space to form whatever it is she wants to say next.

'My friend said I should come because I've been through quite a lot and not really talked about it other than to him.'

'Sounds like you have a good friend looking out for you.'

'Yeah, yeah he is.'

'And you've been through a lot.'

'I didn't think it had impacted me so much but maybe it has.'

'What you've been through has impacted you more than you thought.'

'I think it has yes. I mean I'm through the other side now, but still, when you're going through it, it's like you can't see properly or something, you're just in it.'

'It's difficult to see clearly when you're in the thick of something.'

'Yes, and the process is so fast, you know, there's a system and you just go along with it.'

'The system carries you along.' She half smiles at me as her eyes fill up again and I can feel another burst of emotion erupting. As she opens her mouth to speak, broken words interrupt deep sobs.

'I – had – breast – can – cer.'

'I'm very sorry to hear that, Rosie.' We sit for another few minutes whilst she cries and stops.

'I've not had it as bad as some people, they really go through it.'

'What has it been like for you, Rosie?'

'OK – brutal – but OK. You know it's brutal, there's no other word, but also it was OK.'

'Two extreme tensions you're holding there – brutal and OK.'

'Yeah, it's a strange experience. Like one minute I'm cleaning the kitchen worktop and the next I've found a lump. I thought I'd been bitten – it was hot and I wasn't wearing a bra with my thin summer dress and thought I'd been stung or something. Sounds silly now.'

'Cleaning one minute and the shock of a lump the next.'

'Yeah, and everything just gambolled from there, you know – the doctor, the hospital, scans, biopsy; it was just one appointment to the next. D'you know from start to finish my treatment only took 110 days – that's mad, eh?'

'It felt fast; you gambolled from one appointment to the next.'

'And all the worry in between... although there was hardly any time to worry.'

'You worried.'

Rosie breaks down again, her body shaking as though worry has only just been given voice and expression.

'I didn't worry that I was going to die – well only one night before I saw the GP when I was awake all night and thought *is this it?* You know, the end.'

'You were awake all night worrying if this was the end.'

'I felt soooo awake, it was mad. I sat in the garden at ten o'clock at night and then two o'clock and four o'clock in the morning just listening to the sound of the night, you know... and the smell of summer so strong and I heard the birds waking up, I felt frightened that I was coming to an end and yet I felt more alive than ever in a really weird kind of way.' Like a meerkat, she's upright, eyes wide and animated.

'As you worried about you coming to an end you felt more alive than ever.'

'I did.'

We just rest there in the silence for a moment and I swear I can smell the height of summer and hear birds.

'But my life wasn't really in danger. I mean it was cancer but they said right from the beginning it was treatable, so I just got on with whatever I had to do.'

'Your prognosis was good, the condition treatable and after that night you didn't feel in danger.'

'No, not really. But sometimes a wave of sadness would come over me, like a weird sensation of is this really happening to me, you know?'

'Sadness and questions would wash over you.'

'It was like I was in a movie or was some kind of robot. The minute I got into the hospital I would suddenly lose the power of speech – and I give a lot of speeches, I'm a registrar, you know, weddings, births, services, etc. But I'd get in that hospital and every time the consultant or doctors said something I'd reply "OK" or "OK, thank you". Even when the consultant said I had to have a total mastectomy not a lumpectomy like we first thought. I cried a lot in that appointment, it was such a shock and I wasn't expecting it. I said, "OK, thank you" to the consultant and he said, "You don't need to thank me, I've just given you some not very good news" – the tumour was bigger than they first thought, you see, and in an awkward position,' she is speaking very fast. 'I just said, "Yeah, but you delivered it really well". She sits there looking at me, smiling, seeking confirmation of her strength through humour. I don't flinch.

'You found yourself behaving differently to how you would normally and the situation changed unexpectedly. I notice you seem amused by your loss of the power of speech.'

'I think I was just shocked, out of my depth and just – I dunno – surrendered I suppose. I mean what else can you do in that situation? You have to trust them. I'm sure if the consultant said, "Rosie we're gonna have to take your right leg off as well", I'd have said, "OK, thank you". She laughs and takes a sip of her water.

'You surrendered to the process, a process you knew nothing about and placed your trust in those that did.'

'Yeah.' We sit for a while. I am unfamiliar with treatment for breast cancer so when she says she's through it I don't know what that really means. 'I went through some strange things too. Like I got fixated on buying a kimono – you know – for the hospital.' Her shoulders exaggerate an up-down movement as she chuckles.

'A kimono.'

'I needed a new robe, 'cause I only wear cardis in the summer and my robe is a heavy one for the winter. So, I thought I needed a new one for the hospital. I wanted to feel pretty and nice, so I spent over three hours on the internet one night searching for flowery kimonos. My daughter thought I'd gone mad – she's twenty-two – but it seemed really important to me.' She laughs.

'You wanted to feel pretty and nice as you were about to, what, have surgery? I'm sorry I don't know the treatment process for breast cancer.'

'Oh, sorry, yes, for the mastectomy. I was supposed to only be in for the day but I was poorly, had a bad reaction to anaesthetic, but anyway I still wanted a nice robe, pretty, flowery.'

'Pretty sounds important to you.'

Rosie glares at me and I'm not sure why, she seems speechless and then her eyes fill and her mouth quivers. She glances down at her right breast, which to me looks like a breast and had she not said anything I wouldn't have known about her surgery. Then she looks up at me and through soft wavering words says, 'It's so ugly, brutal – I just wanted something pretty.'

'It feels brutal and ugly to you and you wanted to balance that with some prettiness.'

She raises her hands in the air. 'It's so stupid, I know, stupid.' Tears spit out from her eyes.

'What's stupid?'

'I'm alive – what does it matter I've only got one boob, some people don't have arms or legs, I mean, this doesn't hinder my life really, does it? I mean I've probably lost a few years but in the scale of things, it's been OK.'

'One perspective says it's OK in the scale of things and in another it was brutal, ugly and I notice you have been very sad and distressed telling me about it today, Rosie.' Her eyes fill again.

'My mum used to say that I wasn't pretty – my sister was pretty, she said. My mum said I was attractive. I dunno what that's supposed to mean but you don't say that to a seven-year-old girl, do you? I just wanted pretty things.'

'You were told you were different to your sister and you wanted pretty things.'

'Yeah, a pretty kimono for my ugly surgery. My husband always calls me "his prettiness" – I only just connected those two things.' She looks at me and smiles.

'You've made a connection.' We sit for a moment and I'm wondering what thoughts and images are going through her mind as she considers this connection. I notice how pretty she is; wispy mouse-coloured hair with a golden hue where the sun has caught it, rosy-coloured cheeks and piercing, feline, green eyes; coral toenails peek from under a long skirt made of metres and metres of floral fabric.

'I love my husband, I do, but, because of all this it's made me wonder, you know, what if? What was it all about?'

'Because of your experience through breast cancer you've found yourself with questions.'

'Yeah, we were young, been together forever and now I'm heading towards fifty and he made me feel pretty and now I'm ugly and I know it, you know.'

'You are ugly.'

'I am. He can't look at me. He tries, but he can't. I mean I understand, I couldn't look at first. I couldn't take the dressing off, I left it two weeks for the surgeon to do it.'

'It was difficult for you to look at first and your husband still can't look.'

'How can I still be his... p r e t t i n e s s?' She can barely get the last word out intact. 'I know it's so stupid, I know, I know on the one hand I'm the same person but I'm not and he's not and my son, my son can't talk to me.'

'You feel changed and feel that your relationships with your husband and son have also changed.'

'I know it's hard for them, I know. They're boys, they don't know what to say but it's happened to me,' she puts both hands on her chest, 'to me, it's happened to me.'

'It's happened to you, Rosie.'

She nods and sits still and tears fall silently and more gently. She takes a big breath in and a sip of water from the glass. As she places the glass down she says, 'It's not a man thing though, my friend has been there for me, he can talk and listen to me and I'm sure if I wanted to show him the wound he would look.'

'You have confidence in your friend that he is there for you.'

'Yes – oh there's nothing – I don't want you to get the wrong… he's just a friend, I've known Matt for years, he knows everything about me, you know, he's married, well divorced and with a partner now, but you know, we're good friends.'

'Your friend knows everything about you. Sounds important.'

'Well, I'd never have got through all this without him, he took me to most of my hospital appointments, except the radiotherapy, 'cause Jerry was working – he works in London, and Matt is here and, well, Jerry can't bear it when I'm ill.'

'What's that like for you, that Jerry can't be there for you when you're ill?'

'Oh no, he would, you know, if he could, he's just busy and does that London commute and stuff and, well, I just get on with stuff, it's what we do, how we are, it's OK, but you know…'

'Finish the sentence Rosie, but you know…'

'This was different.'

'Different.'

'I didn't have a cold or something. I had cancer. I still can't believe that when I say it, I had cancer. You'd think he could get over himself for that and be with me.'

'You wanted him with you. I'm curious, Rosie, did you ask him to be with you?'

'What? Erm… no… not really, I mean it's obvious, isn't it, he should've just wanted to be there. It's obvious, isn't it?'

'I really hear how you expected him to just want to be there, but you know, in relationships we have explicit and implicit roles and if you're both used to you just getting on with things as you said earlier, maybe he assumed you'd get on with this too and that you didn't need him.'

'Well I bloody well did need him.'

'How did you communicate that to him?'

'He should've just known, he's not a stupid man.'

'How?'

'It's obvious.'

'And yet it seems that maybe it wasn't so obvious and would've been a real change in the way you behave with one another.'

'Well this was different, there was a change – this was cancer – I could've died – what do I mean to him, really, really what am I to any of them?'

'Who?'

'Everybody: my family, my friends, Jerry, Matt – I dunno – me, what am I to me? What am I now?' Rosie's cheeks go red and whilst her eyes are glazed there is an energy in the air and I would really like to stay with this but am aware we are coming to time.

'What's happened to you is bringing up big questions of what you mean to your family and friends but also to yourself. Who are you? What are you?'

'Yeah, and what do I want?'

'You're also asking what you want.'

'Yes,' she nods a couple of times, 'like what do I want from my life now? Whatever is left, what do I want? I fell in love, got married, had my kids, I work, but really, when did I sit down and ask "is this what I want my life to look like?" Really?'

'Is this what I want my life to look like?'

'Yep.' She's composed in that question and I draw the session to a close, booking in the next one.

Fiona

As I head towards the therapy rooms, I recognise that I don't really want to be there today. I have time to wait for my client so make a cup of tea and sit patiently awaiting her arrival. This room is too big. It needs something more to fill it. Perhaps some foliage. A more substantial floor lamp, as the one in here is thin and not in keeping with the age of the property. It requires something more human with perhaps a warm golden hue rather than the dull silver stem. I must bring in some more artwork for that blank wall. The screen hiding the sink could be more substantial rather than the flimsy pretend Japanese one. What a strange mix of furnishings there are, as though someone threw in all the left-over odds and sods. Still, the three-piece suite helps to make it more of a friendly living room rather than a corporate office. I always forget these thoughts every time I leave the room, and so nothing has changed in five years. I wonder what will unfold in today's session? If the client turns up that is. Fiona doesn't always manage to arrive.

Generally, Fiona's television runs on low volume in the background during the day. Immobilised and constantly feeling chilly, she has described how she sits small, wrapped in a fleecy blanket reminiscing about life, lost moments and missed opportunities until one commercial too many, she will journey her way to the kettle for a cup of tea. Comfortably holding a scalding cup, she will imagine a brisk walk, a routine of busyness, a feeling of energy, making plans, writing, painting, knitting, joining groups, going to church, loving. When she finishes her tea, having momentarily lived, she will feel exhausted and wrap herself up to die once more. This is how Fiona has described her days over the last two months since she has been signed off work. I had felt that Fiona was beginning to improve slightly. She had managed to take a few walks in the park and experienced momentary inspiration from the summer flowerbeds and managed to hold on to the inspiration long enough to pot plants up for her own garden when she got home. Remembering, or being bothered, to water them became a bit of a task, so keeping the momentum was a challenge. Just as Fiona was working on these improvements there came a devastating blow when she informed me last week that her ex-husband had died, suddenly.

Fiona, aged forty-two, is always small in the seat. I think it ironic that she chooses to push herself into the corner of the large sofa rather than take the smaller armchair. As though allowing the large sofa to swallow her. Or perhaps she is too frightened to fill a space fully. She seems insistent upon taking up as little space as possible, and her gentle, yet articulate, voice is always monitored and measured. I have to work hard to maintain my own volume and at the same time be mindful of Fiona's seeming fragility.

'The funeral is on Thursday,' she whispers.

'How is that for you, Fiona, now that you know when it is going to happen?'

'I can't bear it. I want it over and I don't.'

'You do and you don't – sounds like an unbearable tussle going on.'

'I feel that once it's done I might feel better, be able to move somehow, but… I can't… it's too…' Without sound she weeps, her face buried in a tissue held in her hands, shoulders up down, up down. No sound daring to intrude into the air. The box of tissues is on her lap and the bin at her feet. She arranges all this at the beginning of each session. 'I keep replaying that night when he died. The call and the shock and all I kept saying was "not like this, not like this". I just walked in a circle around the room repeating it.'

'"Not like this, not like this", as you circled the room. As you keep replaying that scene is there anything attached to the words – images, colours, sounds, feelings?'

'It's like…' she sobs, 'end… I didn't want…' With great effort, she offers broken words through repeated sobs, and eventually with enough breath to utter the words, 'I didn't want it to end like this.'

I wait a while as Fiona cries through the impact of the words leaving her mouth. I have spent a lot of hours, years, watching people cry. For some, tears fall from the outer edge of the eye. These tears seem to be small, tender, more fragile and quieter than the large voluble globes, which tend to roll on for much longer. Fiona's tears are the only part of her that seems large. As though her tears know how to take their space in a way that the rest of her body just doesn't.

When she settles I offer back, 'You didn't want it to end like this, Fiona.'

She nods her head unable to speak, her mouth covered by scrunched-up tissues in hands making a gag as though she couldn't bear one more word to escape.

We sit silently for some time. The air feels thick with sadness and I find myself drifting off. *What would I do if you died? Who would tell me? What would it make of me? I want to see my eyes reflected back in yours as you breathe your last.* The back of my throat tightens and I swallow down my own imagined grief.

'He kept in touch, you know; nine years apart but he never forgot my birthday. I always got flowers and a message, even at Christmas. I always thought it would end differently.'

'I'm wondering what that meant for you that he kept in touch, particularly on those significant occasions?'

'I know I still mattered. We were a tragedy. I know we still loved each other but he really wanted children and when we realised we couldn't, well I couldn't, then, you know... I've said before...'

'It feels like you were a tragedy and you feel you still loved each other.'

'We did. He said a number of times that he wished it could've been different, he did.'

'What did you take him to mean by that, Fiona?'

'That he wished he'd stayed, that we'd worked it all out.'

'If you had worked it all out and he'd stayed, what do you imagine life would have been like?'

'Happy. We were together at fourteen. I didn't know anyone else. It was always Jason. I can't believe he's gone, I can't believe it, I can't.' Fiona breaks down again and the two of us sit for some time afterwards, silence intermittently broken by deep sobs and the sound of traffic and sirens travelling down the street outside. Fiona doesn't seem to notice. I break the silence, why I don't know – it's unusual for me.

'Fourteen is a very young age, very tender growing years.'

'Yeah, we were just kids, I know, but we never felt like kids. I still feel the same really. We were together fifteen years altogether. He looked after me really, what with my mad brother, and then Dad leaving. Mum never really recovered and just sat in front of the telly eating. I looked after her, and Jason looked after me, it's how it was.' She looks at me with bewildered eyes.

'You were together a long time, sounds like you did a lot of growing-up together too. He was an important support for you when your dad left, he looked after you.'

Almost before I have finished speaking Fiona all but squeals, 'Who is gonna look after me now... what... who?' She verges on the hysterical but is still so tightly bound in the seat that she just holds herself even more tightly as her knees exaggerate their bend in an attempt to pull up. Her feet cannot leave the floor and instead, they come to tiptoe as she folds herself over, taking up less space rather than more. After a few moments she begins to straighten up and she looks at me with the saddest eyes. Like one of those 1970s paintings of children with a globe-like tear about to fall, like a lost child. Like an abandoned child. I wait a moment longer.

'Fiona, I'm aware that I have really strong feelings being with you in such sadness. What I have going on for me is how sad and abandoned you look and sound, and that for a moment you felt like a lost child to me.' The hysterics stop and Fiona looks frightened and glazed eyes stare back at me, almost through me. Gentle tears fall quietly as she continues to stare at me and I feel apprehensive and am now uncertain if my experiential sharing was of any help or whether it has just jarred something for Fiona and taken her away from her own experience.

'What's happening for you as I say that, Fiona?'

'I. I felt. I feel wobbly. I feel like a child. I do feel lost you're right. I am.'

'You are lost.'

'Where am I now he has gone?'

'You don't know where you are now Jason has gone.'

'That sounds mad I know. It's like, even though we weren't together, I knew where he was, and so I knew where I was.'

'Knowing where he was, gave you a sense of your own placing.'

'Where I belonged.'

'You felt you knew where you belonged.'

'Yeah, but I didn't really belong, did I? That's why nobody understands how sad I am. My mum and my friends keep saying "but you weren't together, why are you so sad?"'

'What do you say when they ask you that?'

'I say I don't know. I just am. It just hit me really hard on top of how I was feeling anyway. It's just too much. At least he was there somewhere, and he knew me more than anyone else, more than I knew myself.'

'Losing someone you feel knows you more than you know yourself sounds like a very powerful and immense loss. I can really see how hard it has hit you and impacted your whole sense of belonging. Jason was a big part of your life for a lot of years.'

'Yes, and it's like I'm not supposed to be so sad, but I am.'

I sit back, watch and echo the stillness in Fiona who has momentarily stopped crying. There is something more stable and she seems in command of the faintest moment. Her eyes, though red and puffy, seem not so glazed. She has straightened in her seat and puts tissues in the bin. I don't know why her crying has ceased. All I can do is watch, wait and observe her dazed face as it settles. I wait for Fiona to make her next move and trust that the change in composure is something.

'Maybe I'm sad for me too.'

'You might be sad for you too.'

'I keep imagining him lying on the floor having the heart attack and was he thinking of me. But he was probably thinking of his sons. It must be awful for them. I know my dad didn't die but I know how it feels to lose a dad.'

I notice the time and decide to leave that last statement in the air. It is loaded and requires a deeper exploration than we have time for today. If it matters and means something for Fiona, she will bring it back when she is ready. We agree that our next session will be timely as it will be the day after the funeral and give us an opportunity to be able to work together whilst her experience is still raw.

Felix

'I CAME TO YOU BECAUSE I'M ANXIOUS ALL THE time, I mean aaaallll the time.'

'You experience anxiety at every moment.'

'Yeah, seriously, ALL the time.'

'Are you feeling anxious now?'

'Yeah. I was really scared to come in here.'

'Can you describe your anxiety to me.'

'What… like what it's like?'

'Yes.'

'I dunno… well… it's here.' He places his hands on his belly.

'Is it anywhere else, does it travel?'

He moves his hands over his belly and up towards his throat. 'I guess it's here too.'

'What's the feeling, can you describe it – a colour, shape, temperature?'

'It feels hot, red, but as it gets to my throat it feels tight and burns.'

'It's fiery.'

'Yeah, just like that, like I'm on fire.'

'You feel like you're on fire.'

'Yeah, like I might burst into flames.' His eyes widen and I see an energy in him, like he has come alive in the very expression of his discomfort.

'You might burst into flames. Then what?'

'What d'you mean?'

'What would happen if you burst into flames?'

'I'd die! I mean… I know I won't really burst into flames… but… it feels like that… it's really scary.'

'What's attached to the scared feeling?'

'What d'you mean?'

'Well, what feelings, thoughts, images are swimming around with this scary feeling of anxiety?'

'That everybody's looking at me.'

'Oh, and what are they seeing?'

'I dunno… what d'you mean?' He raises his questioning hands and I detect a little irritation at my questioning style today.

'When you imagine everyone looking at you, what are they seeing, where does your imagination take you?'

'That I don't look right, that I'm stupid… I dunno… that I've got it wrong somehow.'

'You're stupid, look wrong, got it wrong.'

'Yeah.' His eyes are wide as they ask me, *tell me what's wrong, how can I stop the feeling, don't repeat it to me, tell me*. 'It's a horrible feeling, horrible, and I have it all the time, all the time, seriously – all – the time.'

'Yes, I can imagine feeling stupid, looking wrong and getting it wrong is a horrible feeling especially when you have it all the time. Sounds relentless.'

'Well, what do we do… I mean, I don't want the feeling, what can I do to stop it?'

'What have you tried?'

'I've been on anti-depressants for two years now but I'm trying to come off them.'

'Are you consulting with your GP about the dose?'

'Yeah, he's reduced it. I know it has to be done slowly, but I want them out of my system.'

'For what reason?'

'I want to be able to manage and I don't feel like myself taking them. I want to be able to manage.'

'You want to be able to manage and feel like yourself.'

'I don't know if the anxiety is to do with the pills or me, you know, is it who I am? Or are the pills masking who I am? Who am I really?'

'You're not sure if the pills are causing the anxiety or if it is part of you and – if it is part of you – who are you?' He nods, vaguely. 'What's your sense of self right now, who do you feel yourself to be?'

Tears form gently in his young hazel eyes. I watch them build slowly and then, as if they can't remain a moment longer, they leap from the ducts, completely miss his face and drop straight onto his t-shirt, leaving behind an expanding pear-drop.

'Hopeless, I feel hopeless.'

'You feel hopeless.'

'Yeah...' he sobs and raises his hands '... like, what's the point?'

'You're really distressed and asking what's the point?' He nods and cries. I wait.

Felix is young, twenty years old. He explained in his email to me that he's a student at the university here, not English and yet his English is better than mine. He's already lived in six different countries, been to different schools all over the world, was born in Canada but hasn't lived there since the age of two. His parents currently live in South Africa, but he considers home to be in France where he spent his early years, and where his grandmother still lives.

'When you ask what's the point, Felix, what do you mean?'

'Like, what's the point of being here if I just feel like this all the time?'

'Being here meaning?'

'Alive, what's the point?'

'What's the point of living if you feel like this all of the time?'

'Yeah.'

'It's a good question, so what keeps you here?'

'Huh?'

'You're very distressed, feel horribly anxious all of the time, think that people are judging you as stupid and wrong. I'm curious what keeps you here when you feel like that.'

'Well I can't just... I mean I've thought about it... but... it would kill my parents, and my little brother, I mean it would devastate them, if I, you know, did anything.'

'Your family would be devastated. Sounds like your family is really important to you.' Quietly, he nods.

'They are. I miss them, all the time. I'm used to being away, but I miss them. I go back to see my granny in Paris as much as I can.'

'You like to spend time with your granny as much as possible.'

'Yeah, that's more my home than anywhere.'

'Where granny is feels like home for you.'

'Yeah, I first went to school in Paris and she looked after me and my brother because my mum and dad worked a lot. She's so sweet and funny and the house always smells of bakery – she's always making things, she's warm. I just love her.' More tears fall from his face forming an irregular mottled pattern on the thin blue marl t-shirt. He seems oblivious to their landing. 'She's not very well.'

'Your granny is unwell.'

Felix nods as he sobs and his shoulders shake.

'I'm sorry to hear that, Felix.'

'They think she's had a stroke. I don't know all the details, I'm going to Paris this afternoon.'

'That all sounds very sudden and uncertain. How are you feeling about going this afternoon?'

'I can't wait, I just really want to be there, see her, know she's alright… but… what if… what if she's not? What if she doesn't re-' *sob* '-cover?' He sits and cries into a hand full of tissues, hiding his face. I feel myself wince. This is very painful for him. I'm reminded of my own daughter's grief when her granny died. All I wanted to do was hold her tight for as many years as it would take for the pain to subside as though I were the only thing that could help. An arrogance easing my own pain.

'I'm sorry, I'm just really scared. I don't want her to die.'

'You're close to her and scared that she might die.'

'Yeah, closer than anyone, and she's so funny, she doesn't get all the technology, you know, she says we should all develop technophobia and eat cake and the world would be much better off.' Felix giggles and snorts up some snot. 'I think she gets it really but she says I worry too much. I talk to her on the phone once a week and visit as much as I can. It's always good to be there.'

'Feels good to be in her company and keep regular contact. What is it that she thinks you worry about?'

'What I said earlier really, that I'm not good enough.'

'You don't feel good enough.'

'No.'

'In what context do you feel that?'

'Every context – all the time.'

'OK, give me an example of when it feels strongest.'

'Erm, in lectures – or when, you know, I'm out with friends.' I'm always amazed by how many people come to therapy because they feel anxious with their friends. I would love a whole group of friends to come to therapy so they can all be honest about their insecurities and projections and work it all out.

'You're a student so I guess you have a lot of lectures and you're young so I'm imagining you go out a lot with friends too.'

He laughs. Maybe I suddenly feel like funny granny to him.

'Yeah, but sometimes I miss a lecture and pretend I'm busy so I don't have to go out.'

'Sometimes you avoid situations that make you anxious.'

'Yeah, and my friends are good, I think they know really but they say "just do what you gotta do", you know, they're good like that.'

'You feel you have supportive friends.'

'Yes, but I feel I let them down.'

'How so?'

'By making excuses for not going out sometimes. I think they must get sick of me.'

'Why would they be sick of you?'

'Because, I'm weak – it's weak to just keep giving in to the anxiety, but it's so hard you know, it's so hard.' Felix stares down at the bunch of damp squidged tissues in his hands. He turns them over and over as if they were a crystal ball.

'It feels weak to be anxious? Sounds a little harsh on yourself given that anxiety is a part of life. I'm wondering in what situations d'you think anxiety is not weak, Felix?'

'Oh, I dunno – bungy jumping or skydiving, or being on an island with Bear Grylls.' He smirks.

'What's different about anxiety in those situations?'

'Well, you could die – you know – fall, crash to the earth or starve and die.'

'How do you feel about death, Felix?' As he breaks down into energetic sobs, I feel maybe my question was too real, and asked all too soon. He is, after all, frightened enough right now. As he starts to settle, I say, 'My question seemed to really upset you.'

'It shocked me… I think it frightened me.'

'You felt frightened, Felix.'

'Yeah.'

'What does fear feel like for you in your body – where did you feel it?'

'Right here,' he places his hands on his stomach once more, 'like when I feel anxious like I said before, but it's not red, it was black – empty – black.'

'When I asked how you felt about death you felt a sensation of black emptiness in your body.'

'I don't want my granny to fall into black emptiness.'

'You're frightened that your granny is going to die and it will be a black emptiness.' He just nods.

'I know we all die, and she is old, but I'm not ready.'

'Yes, I really hear that, Felix, I really hear and see in you that you're not ready for that.'

We sit in more silence for a few moments as sadness looms in the air. Whenever we come into contact with death, we also come into contact with life. When we speak of not wanting to be here, we are articulating what it feels to be here. And in all that exploration, possibilities can arise. He looks at his watch, then at his phone, then at me.

'What time are you travelling?' I ask.

'I'm going to the station when I leave here.' In this response, I realise we are finished for today and somewhere in his psyche Felix is already travelling to Paris. We arrange our next appointment and I wish him a good journey. It is all I can do.

Meg

'It's been a very hard week. I haven't slept well and everyone at work seems to have triggered my sadness. I thought I was alright but then… well this week made me realise I'm not.'

'You're sadness has been triggered at work this week.'

'Yeah, I dunno, it's not work, it's just too many buttons pushed and I just feel like I need to do something.'

'You need to take action somehow.'

'Yes, unlike my mother who just lay and wallowed.'

'You compare yourself to your mother.'

'I guess she's never far away.'

'It feels as though she is close to you.'

'It maddens me when I hear myself say these things.'

'You feel mad with yourself when you speak of your mother in this way.'

'I do. Why can't I just leave her behind? What am I holding on to exactly?' I keep eye contact, not hearing the question as one for me to answer. 'I suppose I've just always been so determined not to live the way she did. I always take steps in the opposite direction.'

'You keep hold of your mother by taking steps in the opposite direction.'

'I refuse to hold on so tightly as she did to the fantasy of a man who was not there. And her refusal to let it go and live out her life in a more productive way could've brought her so much happiness instead of the misery she inflicted upon herself, and me.'

'It was miserable for you.'

'Yes, not knowing what I was going to be waking up to, and … well … no not always. I was taken care of by my aunt and uncle and had a normal childhood really, and mum could be funny when she wasn't howling. I was determined to be a different kind of mother to my own children.'

'How many do you have?'

'Two, Jenny and Mathew. In their thirties now. They've both done well, good careers and stuff. They both have two children too, so I'm a granny and that makes me happy.' She looks up at me and smiles. 'I wish they'd have been more bohemian though.'

'In what way?'

'Oh I dunno, I'm being mean, they've done really well and have secure jobs in teaching and accounting but… I just wanted more for them.'

'You feel mean saying it but wanted more for them somehow.'

'I wanted them to be artists, travellers or explorers – or something romantic like poets or musicians – they were free and had such opportunity.'

'You speak as though they have missed opportunities or are... mmm... I dunno, are trapped maybe, no longer free?'

'I know. It's not what I mean and they've done really well: secure marriages, lovely families, holiday homes, I'm proud, I am.'

'And yet you sound deflated somehow.'

'I know. It's not about them. It's me. I'm deflated. They really enjoy their lives. Nothing really seems to trouble them. They seem stable. How do they stick at it?'

'How they manage their lives eludes you.' Her eyes begin to fill.

'It does. I didn't want to be a divorced woman and I didn't want that for my children but I just couldn't stay.'

'You also said in a previous session that it was the right thing for you at the time.'

'Yes, I know. And in the long-run it is too, probably. We're so different, Richard and me. He needed someone who doesn't really have anything to say... I dunno, not restless like me.'

'You're restless.'

'Always, I think.' She drops her head and watches her fingers as they twiddle. 'Except when I was with Len.'

'You didn't feel restless with Len.'

'No. Everything was there, in its place. I felt, I dunno, right – it all felt right, like I was in the right place. Yes I was at home... within myself.'

'When you were with Len you felt at home within yourself. What does home feel like, Meg?'

'Safe, warm, easy, lovely.'

'Safe, warm, easy and lovely. Sounds idyllic.'

'It was. It was my ideal relationship. No drudgery, dependency.'

'It was your ideal relationship, all the highs, none of the lows, none of the ordinariness like the lives of your children.'

'You think it wasn't real because we only had the highs.'

'Why would I think that?'

'Because it's a question I constantly ask myself. But you know, we argued sometimes too and I would feel rejected when he spoke of his happy marriage. I didn't want to know. I just wanted to be in the space that we had created; the spaces where we met.'

'You didn't want your space to be spoiled.'

'It wasn't just hotel rooms for the afternoon. Sometimes we'd go away to other counties, other countries a few times too. Those occasions were bliss.'

'What was blissful about them?'

'It was as though the world had fallen away and there was just us because we were anonymous to the world. There were no intrusions.'

'Anonymity and no intrusions… of ordinary life?'

'I suppose. Was it just a fantasy? Really, have I deluded myself? I always felt that my children's lives were a fantasy, a delusion – I keep waiting for them to wake up really.'

'Maybe however we design our lives they're all fantasy.'

'Well everything felt real enough this week.'

'How d'you mean?'

'I couldn't bear the feelings. I just couldn't quell them so I decided to pay him a visit.'

'You went to see Len?'

'It was a spur of the moment thing but yes, I was angry and frustrated and wanted to see his reaction if I turned up at his house.'

'You went to his house?' I notice my stomach surge.

'I stood on the corner and waited. I sort of felt unwell and I was angry like, how dare he treat me like this? I am not nothing. I am something. Something! Why would he cause me so much pain, why? ME of all people, why would he do that to ME? I kept having this argument with myself about telling his wife so that she can make the decision, I mean she has no choice if she doesn't know.'

'You are something and were in an argument with yourself and all those contradictory answers.'

'Yeah, I guess. I was so confused… lashing out but couldn't seem to stop myself and then just as I talked myself into leaving he came around the corner arm-in-arm with his wife. They were meandering, chatting, just as he'd done with me loads of times. I felt breathless and frozen. I couldn't move my feet and just watched. He looked up at me and smiled but carried on walking like I made no impact. I didn't know how to behave. I cried and could hear a little voice saying, *see my pain, see my pain.* But they carried on walking to the front door. He closed the door. I wanted my legs to just give way so that I could fall to the ground. Cause a scene.'

'See my pain, see my pain. You wanted to have an impact and show how bereft you felt.'

'I felt bereft and I wanted him to see how bad it felt for me. I was just about to leave when he opened the door and just stood looking at me. He put his hand up and gently nodded his head with a half-smile before closing it again.' She sits with silent tears running down her cheeks. I'm aware of the journey my own gut has just travelled as I listened to this description of heartbreak. I notice I feel relieved that she hadn't exposed her lover. I'm unsure what that is about. Is it that I feel something significant must survive, that whatever it was that they had shared for twenty years must be allowed to live and if she had exposed it something would have died? Yes, love must be left to linger intact, in the ether of all existence. Even if without us around to witness it. Tess springs to mind. Her agony at her loss, even now after all this time, as she approaches her own death.

'I seemed to be in a daze when I got back home and went to bed in my clothes – I couldn't get warm.'

'I'm not surprised; it sounds like it was a very draining experience.'

'It was. I woke up at 3am drenched and delirious. I looked around the bedroom and thought *what now?*'

'What answer did you come up with?'

'I didn't. I just wandered around the house with the dog, looking at all my books. They're all about us you see, me and him, what we shared. Books forming our history. It was like looking at a wall of belonging. But it suddenly felt too high, overbearing, and I felt closed in and suffocated. So I took books off the shelves and started stacking them like dismantling bricks from a wall.'

'You dismantled your history.'

'Yeah, I will take it to Oxfam.'

I notice I feel myself wince. It feels too soon to be sorting through the dearly departed belongings. But who am I to know what is too soon? *For sure I'm not ready to dismantle you.*

'What d'you think your activity gave you in that moment?'

'I know what you're thinking.'

'What am I thinking?'

'That I'm just reacting against my mother and refusing to play the dying swan.'

'What do you feel about that thought?'

'That it's probably right; it's a game to get me through, but I don't care, I have to get through as best I can.'

'You feel you're playing a game with yourself and against your mother as a process through your grief.'

'Mmm, and also I think I was angry and wanted to wipe him out. Spite him somehow by discarding what was special to us. I want him to feel discarded, like I do.'

'You feel discarded.'

'I do. I know it's stupid but I do.'

'The unavailable man, discarded you.'

'Why do you keep using that phrase? It really fucks me off.'

'Why does it fuck you off?'

'Because,' she shuffles in her seat, 'because, well, I feel you judging me, like it's my own fault 'cause he was never available in the first place.'

'Is that maybe how you feel about yourself?'

She breaks down and all but screeches, 'I've played everything wrong all along, all my life, I got it wrong.' She buries her head in her hands.

'You got it all wrong, Meg?'

She nods as she speaks, 'I thought I always had to fight, to not give in like her but I caused myself so much pain. Why couldn't I just be still like her, stay put.'

'Stay put where?'

'With Richard and my children, just see it through.'

'Because at the time you couldn't, you have stated repeatedly that you just couldn't.'

'Yes. Yes, I know. I know, but it all hurts so much.'

'Yes, I see how it hurts, Meg.' We sit silently for what seems like quite a few minutes and I feel a few tugs at my own scars of loss that are left on my heart; my lover's face flashing up before me. After a while she looks up at me, face a little lighter, eyes a little drier.

'The day after that I went to my daughter's house for the twins' birthday party – they're five.' I smile having no idea where this is going; we seem to have changed track suddenly. 'Richard was there of course, with his wife. We exchanged a few words, we're friendly, but you know in truth, I was irritated. He had nothing to say; we don't really have anything in common. So you see, in the end, I didn't make a mistake even though sometimes life feels very hard.'

'You feel it was the right decision for you and your life even though it is hard sometimes.'

'I do, it's just sometimes, when life feels hard I wonder *what if,* you know? Could I have made it easier somehow? I know life is just hard sometimes and in truth… I wouldn't have missed out on what I've had so far.'

I say nothing, and just look at her red damp face. I want to say, *Yes! It's really fucking hard.* And I want to be glib and say, *It is what it is in any given moment and will pass.* She breaks the ponder-filled air. 'I will be away for the next two weeks as I have decided to go away and just have some time away to think about all this.'

We agree to meet the week after her return.

Luke

LUKE STARES INTO SPACE FOR SOME TIME. I WATCH.

'I just want something to happen,' he states quietly, without moving a muscle.

'I notice how still you are as you say that, Luke. It felt very passive to me.'

'Passive, what d'you mean passive?' He looks alert.

'Now you sound a little cross. What I meant was that you said "I want something to happen" but it felt said without energy, like you are just waiting for something *to* happen to you. I experienced it as a kind of passivity... or... powerlessness maybe is a better word.'

'Oh, I see, yeah, well I feel powerless.'

'What is it that you feel powerless about?'

'Making something happen – I just said.'

'You sound irritated or something.'

'I am. Everybody wants a piece of me.'

'Everybody wants a piece of you, like you are a thing.'

'Exactly like that. I feel like a thing divided up between people for their own benefit.'

'You are a thing divided up between people. What people?'

'Cherry and the kids, work, Rebecca, my in-laws. Everybody wants a piece of me.'

'You feel like a thing that everybody wants a piece of. And we know that you are not a thing.'

'Yeah, but it feeeeels like that.' Luke sits up and leans forward, and he has turned up the volume of his voice, gritted his teeth, and his face is stony as he stares at me, leaving his statement in the air. I waste no time and respond on the rise.

'I really noticed the energy rise in you then, and I felt my own energy rise too.'

'Why? Why is your energy rising?'

'Because I guess I enjoyed experiencing your energy – it felt active.'

'You want me to be active?'

'I don't want you to be anything, I'm merely sharing my own experience of what I observed in you.'

'Well, this isn't about you, it's about me.'

'Yes, it's about you. My sharing that I noticed your energy rise wasn't helpful to you?'

'Nope.'

'I'm sorry, my intention for it was to be helpful. I guess I'm not a thing either and so I get things wrong sometimes and I really want to be helpful.'

'You can't help though, can you? I mean we go round and round but nothing actually happens?'

'You'd like something to happen?'

'Well, isn't that the point? I've been coming here for a long time now and yes it helped in the beginning and things changed but it doesn't seem to do much now.'

'Therapy isn't doing much for you now and you'd like it to help you make something happen.'

'And I'm sick of you repeating everything.'

'You sound really exasperated, Luke.'

'I am *aarrgh*.'

We sit in silence for quite a while but I am liking the energy in the room and I feel awake.

I decide to surrender and wait for his next move in this dance. I wish he would just say what he needs to say. The air is thick with possibility of a sentence. I can sit this out for the full fifty minutes if need be. For his sake, because if he can bring himself to say the words, and hear himself, experience in his own body the impact of his own audible words, then he may be able to move, shift in some way. Of course, he may not have the words. That's the thing about the unconscious: it doesn't know what it is – yet.

'I just want everybody to fuck off.'

'You want everybody to fuck off. Is there a pecking order of who you'd like to fuck off first?'

'Oh yeah Rebecca, no Cherry... I... *arrgh*... I dunno.' He makes a big movement in his seat as if he is going to stand. Instead he puts one leg under the other and sits on it.

'Luke, you don't have to sit there confined to the seat, move around the room if you want to – stand up.'

Alarmed, his eyes stare back at me. I want to stand up, to show him and say *look here is how you can move*, but I know he knows how to stand, to walk, to have control over his own movement. I want to treat him like a child and demonstrate, like a mother would, how to stand up in the world. Luke breaks the tension, shuffles some more in his seat and a gentle, if not snide, chuckle leaves his mouth.

'I don't have to get up.'

'No, you don't and yet I also heard today how you want something to happen.'

'Well standing up and going walkabout in here won't make anything happen.'

'Is there anything that you feel you can do to make something happen?'

'Yeah, I need to make a decision.'

'You need to make a decision.'

He sits forward and puts his elbows on his knees and places his hands together in a kind of prayer position. As he keeps his head bowed over his praying hands, his eyes look up at me and his head nods.

'I love Cherry and the kids, I really do and it is killing me knowing what I am doing could smash everything up. I don't want that for them, or me actually.' His eyes fill.

'You don't want to smash everything up for any of you.'

'Nope. Rebecca is pushing really hard for me to do that, though.'

'You feel pushed.'

'Don't get me wrong, she's a good person and I know she loves me and we have a great time but it's not real life, is it? Cherry and the kids, school, her parents, all the crap

– I mean that's real life, isn't it?' He sits back into the seat and rests his hands on his belly. I wish people wouldn't add "real life" to their statements as though there is such a thing.

'Are you asking me or telling me?'

'Both – nah, I know it really. I know that Cherry knows. I caught her crying the other day, she said it was just hormones or something. We both pretended it was about her mum being ill and stuff but there was a look in her eye, something in the air, I dunno, I'm just sure she knows and I can't bear it.'

'You can't bear that she knows.'

'I can't bear what it is doing to her, it kills me.' We sit for a few moments in the killing atmosphere. Silence is a powerful activity where the moment of experience can be known if we listen carefully as the air whispers above, below and within. 'I have to make a decision – I have to end it with Rebecca.'

I respond with a deliberate unfluctuating tone, 'Your decision is to end it with Rebecca.'

'I have to, it can't go on like this. I can't give her what she wants because I'm never going to leave Cherry and I can't carry on living in this torment. None of us can.' I stay still and silent, leaving the words ringing in the air, not wanting to reinforce or contradict them in any way. We sit for some time digesting the statement. I can feel his torment. The curdling of all his feelings, values and desires. It is a waiting game. A baking game.

Luke glances at the clock and then back at me. 'I don't think I have anything else to say…'

'We have ten minutes left, Luke. Is it worth using the time to explore how you're feeling now that you have articulated your decision?'

'No. I'm done for today. I just wanna go I think.'

'OK, Luke.' I pick up my diary and, feeling his vulnerability, I ask without lifting my head, 'where you off to when you leave here?'

'I'll go and sit in the park for a bit before I go home. Sam's got tennis practice and I said I'd pick him up.'

I nod an acknowledgement of having heard that he wants to go. 'OK, alright for next week?'

'Yeah, that's fine. Sorry about getting arsy with you. It just feels like a lot, you know.'

Luke leaves behind a heaviness in the air – an anger. Loss produces such anger for us but in that there can be great energy. His decision looms as he now has to find a way of acting upon it.

Rosie

'I HAD A BIG ROW WITH JERRY AFTER I LEFT HERE last time.'

'You did?'

'Yeah, I just wanted to know why he kept going to work.'

'You had some questions that you wanted answers to.'

'He said he thought I was OK, that I was dealing with things and carried on, that he didn't want to interfere. I told him I felt let down.'

'You felt let down by Jerry.'

'Yes, well, no, not at the time but now, I feel let down now. I did just get on with things, I did, I know I did, it's what I do. We talked about that, how we are, but, now, you know it's different.'

'It feels different now.'

'I feel different. I just want... want, oh I dunno, I'm not the same.'

'You don't feel the same and you want.'

'How can I be the same after this? How can I go back to how things were before? Everything is so different now.'

'Everything feels different.'

'Yeah.' We sit silently for a while as she mulls something over in her mind whilst she twizzles a tissue between her fingers – looping the loop – and I wonder what thoughts and feelings are looping the loop for her right now. 'It's weird, I know I'm different but I can't put my finger on what it is 'cause in another sense I'm not different.'

'Feels weird to be different and not different; changed and not changed.'

'Yes, that's more like it, something has changed obviously...' She looks down at her right breast. '...But also somethings have not changed.' A fire engine screeches past the window on its way to a situation of change no doubt. 'I know my body has changed but I seem to be able to cope with that alright. Sometimes it's ugly but at other times I just put the prosthesis in my bra and feel fine. It's strange when I turn over in bed and don't have to drag the other boob with me. Actually, it's quite freeing not having boobs I think. But I do prefer to have the boob in if I have to go out.'

'Your body has changed and there seems to be some benefit to not having a boob but if you're going out you prefer to have it.'

'Mmmm, I like to look nice and I don't really want people I don't know knowing what I've been through.'

'It's private.'

'Yes, you know, it is private. I like that. Private. It happened to me, was mine in a way.'

'I'm wondering if maybe Jerry picked that up from you somehow.'

'What d'you mean?'

'Well, I dunno, maybe somehow you communicated through the way that you relate to one another that this was your journey, your experience.'

'I shut him out you mean?' She sounds defensive.

'Not necessarily and I don't mean to suggest on purpose if you did, just that perhaps you are so self-sufficient in your marriage that as you said earlier you "get on with it".'

'Hmmm, yeah maybe. But then I did share it all with Matt so I didn't want to get on with it by myself.'

'What is it about Matt that you felt you could share with him in a way that you couldn't with your husband?'

'I don't know. We've known each other a long time... and... well... I spend more time with him I guess and I know all about his marriage and relationships, all the ins and outs.'

'You are his confidante.'

'I suppose I am really.'

'He shares with you.'

'Yeah, he shares, I don't have to ask, with Jerry it's like pulling teeth.'

'Matt volunteers information, Jerry has to be asked.'

'Yeah, and even then I don't always get an answer.'

'So you are left in the dark sometimes.'

'Yes! Exactly that. It's like I don't really know what's going on in him. Don't get me wrong, he's the kindest man and we have a good marriage but it's like I can't reach him.'

'Or feel reached yourself.' She stares at me.

'I want to feel... oh I don't know... something... alive, you know? I want to feel alive, like I did that night sat in the garden crying, thinking this was the end.'

'You don't feel so alive as you did that night.'

'No, there was a real energy and even in the dark the colours as the sun came up were so... so... sharp and vibrant.'

'As though the scene came alive for you.'

'Yes.'

'And what's your scene now, Rosie?'

'That's what I mean, it's the same, even though I feel different, everything is the same, going back to normal, quite dull really.'

'The scene of your life feels dull.'

'Yes – no – oh not all of it I mean – God – just is there more?'

'Is there more?'

'Well, do I just carry on with my job and my family? The kids, they've practically left home, my daughter is twenty-two and working; my son is nineteen at university. Jerry'll be doing what he does 'til he retires, but what about me, what about me now?'

'What about you now?'

'I've had this mad idea for years – well everybody thinks it's mad, the kids roll their eyes and Jerry doesn't say anything.' I say nothing, waiting to see if she can tell me what her mad idea is. She looks at me and I can feel her wanting me to ask, pulling an invisible thread between us. 'It's a bit mad but I think it could work, and I've had the idea for so long.'

'You've had the idea for a long time.'

'Yeah, and it's you know, not far from what I do now really but more, well, independent and exciting, and it wouldn't be here in this bloody East Anglian flatland, it would mean a move.'

'It would mean a move, a different landscape, and is similar to what you do now.'

'Yeah, well, you see, I love Cumbria, you know the Lake District?' I nod. 'We've had loads of holidays there and I just love it and I know, I know it's a cliché but I've always wanted to run a tea shop.' She stares at me intensely trying to catch a glimpse of disapproval, approval, or judgement of any kind. 'Everyone rolls their eyes and says how hard work it is like I don't know that.' We sit a while and I don't take my eyes off her. 'Well, my idea is that we run a tea shop but you have to have something extra as well. I'm a registrar and could offer ceremonies and services, like a celebrant; quirky tea shop weddings, christenings or anniversaries, hand-fastening and the retaking of vows.' We sit some more, looking at each other, me with an image of flowers and cupcakes and a smell of baking up my nostrils. 'I think it could work, it's quirky I know but…' She awaits my response.

'But?'

'It's mad, I know.' And she deflates into her seat.

'Why mad, Rosie?'

'Because it'd mean giving everything up and moving and starting again and it might not work and… and… I dunno… I can't do it on my own.'

'What d'you need?'

'What d'you mean?'

'You said you can't do it on your own, so what or who do you need?'

'Well, the kids, they're still at home and…' She raises her hands in the air as if the ether confirms her thoughts.

'You said earlier the kids have all but gone, your daughter works and your son is at university.'

'Yes, but they wouldn't want to go to Cumbria, and Jerry, I mean I need him to be with me, I'd like him to want to be there too.'

'Have you spoken to the family about it?'

'Yes – well no, not exactly, I mean I make little jokes about it and they makes jokes about it.'

'Your idea is a joke between you all.'

'No, yes, I mean… hmmm…' Her eyes fill up.

'What's happening now, Rosie, as your eyes fill up?'

'Nobody takes me seriously.'

'You don't feel taken seriously.'

'No, but then, maybe I haven't taken it seriously either. Maybe I don't really think it can be possible and it's just a pipe dream.'

'It might be a pipe dream, Rosie, if it is then what?' Tears stream down her face gently and quietly.

'Then…' she raises her hands skyward again '…then this is it, this is my life.'

'Nothing changes.'

'Exactly, nothing changes and then what's it all been for?'

'What's it all been for – what are you referring to?'

'The cancer, it must be for something. I can't have gone through all this for nothing; it must matter, make a difference somehow.'

'The cancer must count for something.'

'Yes! Yes, I can't go back to how things were, I can do something different.'

'What I really hear from you, Rosie, is that whilst you have been through great change physically and emotionally you are craving some, I don't know, practical kind of change too, that would what – what would that change give you?'

'Life: I'd feel alive.'

'You want to feel alive and you have an idea that neither you nor your family really take too seriously, but which might help you to have that feeling of aliveness.'

Rosie sits quietly and nods, bowing her head as she does so. She looks around the room and picks up a cushion from the sofa she is sitting on.

'You see this fabric? Did you pick the cushion, is it yours?'

'No, it belongs to the centre.'

'At the hospital when they tell you all about the surgery, they give you a bag, like a school swimming bag, you know with the drawstring?' I nod. 'It's pink, obviously, and in it is your temporary prosthetic, a leaflet, the NHS issue bra and a cushion. The cushion is heart-shaped. But it's pointy – not a rounded heart, it's a pointy heart.' I listen with intent having no idea where this is going. 'I hated it when I first saw it, the shape of it but mostly the fabric. It's horrid, isn't it? Cheap fabric and I loathe the colours, it's not me at all.'

'The cushion wasn't a match for you in so many ways.'

'Yeah. I spent ages looking at what scraps of fabric I had to recover it. They said I should take it to the hospital with me when I go for surgery – take everything just in case they said. It's for under the arm you see, 'cause your boob acts as a kind of spacer between the chest wall and your arm. Well anyway, I took it. The worst part of the surgery is under the arm where they take the lymph nodes from. I was swollen for weeks and my arm was two inches shorter than it used to be – honest – it was so painful, sore and uncomfortable. Anyway, it turned out that the cushion was a godsend. It helped cushion the soreness, created space between my arm and my side and kinda folded in front because of the pointy shape, like a boob.'

'The cushion became so many things for you and it became more important than you thought it would be.'

'Yeah, but when I got home, in bed I had to sleep almost upright for a while, so Jerry slept in the spare room. When he came back, I could still only sleep on my back and fairly upright for quite a while. Eventually I could lie on my left side with the cushion under my right arm still. It took a couple of months before I could turn on to my right side, which is where Jerry sleeps. And he couldn't roll over towards me because the cushion was in the way and I was sore, and I think he was frightened.'

'It's as though you were sleeping separately even though you were in the same bed, with your back to each other.'

'Yeah, and we never slept like that before, and I just realised looking at this cushion, that I still sleep with the cushion.' Rosie pummels the cushion, smooths it out and then pummels it again.

'What does it mean for you, Rosie, that you still sleep with the cushion?' Her eyes tear up.

'I think it's like a comforter. I hold on to it for dear life sometimes...' She has a good, long cry, holding the cushion tightly and close to her body. 'I miss it... my breast... I miss it and sometimes feel so sad and my husband can't get near because I hold the cushion in the way.'

I don't feel any need to respond to this other than allow my eyes to fill as hers have done so. It is sad. After a few moments she puts the cushion back, straightening it out and takes a tissue to blow into.

'Maybe I miss my husband too.'

'You miss Jerry.'

'I do. Everything is so different and I know he doesn't know how to respond. I haven't known how to be but I guess I've been in it and just swept along.'

'It's been difficult for both of you to know how to be with one another and it sounds like you're saying you had no time to really think about it as you were the one being swept along by the process of it all.'

'Yeah, maybe we need to talk about it. I think I've been angry with him and I don't know why.'

'You've been angry at Jerry.'

'Yes, not intentionally, but you know, I just felt my life getting out of control, slipping away and I think I expected him to do something, but, really, there was nothing for him to do, and in any case, he kept the family going, he did, he did keep going for us.'

'It felt like life was out of control for you, Rosie, slipping away and in the background Jerry kept things going.'

'Yeah, like life as I knew it was slipping away and I didn't know where I'd end up. And... I'm ashamed to say I don't think I even noticed Jerry.'

'You didn't know what the end would be and lost sight of Jerry.'

'But also I did, I mean they said from the outset "this is treatable", it's not like my life was really in danger even though it was cancer, but I knew I would just go back to work and get on with things again but I didn't... I didn't expect to feel that I didn't want to go back to it.' We're back to work and identity and have lost Jerry again.

'You imagined things to go back to how they were but find yourself not wanting that.'

'Yeah, I want something different, not sure what, but something, and I realise I've been really hard on Jerry whilst I've been feeling this way. He must've felt shut out.' Rosie seems to rest herself in the statement and my response is to be silent and let the words linger in the air and sink in, it feels like an important articulation.

I notice the time and we arrange our next appointment.

Felix

FELIX TAKES HIS SEAT AFTER SOMEWHAT SHUFFLING into the room. He looks dishevelled, tired; eyes dark with a red tinge as though someone had pencilled in crimson eyeliner.

'You look tired, Felix.' His eyes glaze with water and remain glass-like as he nods.

'I haven't slept too well, only got back yesterday.' He stares at me momentarily. 'My granny is OK and home now.' I notice myself relax as I was poised to hear that she had passed.

'How do you feel about her being at home?'

'My mum is there, but they don't really get on and I didn't really want to leave and come back.'

'You didn't want to come back.'

'No, I wanted to stay and look after her but Mum was insistent.'

'Mum insisted you come back.'

Nodding he stares down at the floor. 'Yeah, she never really listens to me.'

'You don't feel listened to.'

'Nope.' As he stares at the floor once more, I see a tension in his face. His young beard looks a little bristled and the moment feels a little charged. I wait it out, aware that in my last session with him I asked a lot of questions. Maybe he needed the questions from me and I felt him pulling them to help structure his session. But if he can talk without me interrogating him then he's got a better chance of being heard, and it seems like he's not getting that from home right now.

'I didn't want to come here.'

'Therapy? You didn't want to come today?'

'No, Cambridge. I didn't want to come to Cambridge. I wanted to stay in Paris.'

'D'you mean you didn't want to be at university or do you mean the city? You wanted to be in Paris.'

'Both. I don't like it here.'

'What made you decide to come?'

'It's Cambridge! My parents were ecstatic and said I should come as I'd been offered a place. Everyone said I should come. I mean it's the best, right?'

'Depends what you mean by "the best" I guess; best for what, for who?'

'Education. I mean it's like a golden ticket, you know, to get a job.'

'It's a golden ticket to a job.'

'Well that's what they think, my parents, but that's 'cause they work all the time. I don't want that.'

'Working all the time is not for you.'

'No, yeah, I mean...' He shuffles in his seat, bowing his head as he does so and adjusts his jumper, running his hands through a mass of wavy strawberry-blond hair. He looks up at me when he has become still again. 'I mean I know I have to work, but you know, it seems all I've done is be at school and I have to choose what to do next year and they want me to stay and do my Masters.'

'*They* being?'

'My teachers and parents. I know it's probably the best decision, but I don't think it's what I want.'

'You might want something different.'

'Yeah.' A big grin comes across his face.

'I'm not sure if your grinning is happiness, hope or cheeky defiance.'

He lets out a chuckle and looks me straight in the eye. 'All three I think.'

'Your energy has risen and you feel happy, hopeful and defiant with your grin.'

We sit for a moment in the quiet and a fire engine screeches past keeping the energetic momentum.

'I'm curious what thoughts or images are attached to the feelings of happy, hopeful and defiance, Felix. Like, what do you imagine for yourself that ignites such feelings?'

'You'll laugh if I tell you.' He grins, testing my response to his obvious vulnerability.

'You feel that you know what I am thinking and feeling.'

'NO! I mean no, but you know, everybody laughs.'

'Other people laugh when you tell them so you feel I might laugh too.'

'Yeah.'

'And if I do laugh, what then? Because I can't promise that I won't, I mean I have no idea how I will feel until the feeling comes up. I guess it's hard to say it to me knowing that you've already experienced being laughed at.'

'I don't think they're laughing at me, I think maybe they just want what's best for me.'

'Who are you speaking about when you say "they"?'

'My parents, mainly.'

'Your parents laugh at you.'

'Sounds bad, it's like a laugh but they glance at each other, like they know... I feel, I dunno, put down a bit, like I'm too young to know my own mind, which is annoying 'cause most of the time I'm left in different countries to just get on with it.'

'It feels confusing to be left to get on with things and then feel a little, I don't know, ridiculed a bit by knowing glances.'

'Yeah, exactly that, I'm really confused.'

'You're confused.'

'Yeah, like should I stay and finish my degree and stay for my Masters, or just, you know...'

'Just? Finish the sentence, Felix.'

'Just go to Paris and, you know, just live.'

'Your other option is to go and live in Paris.'

'Yeah.'

'What would you do there? What's the image of your life in Paris?'

'I'd be by my granny, I'd get a job in a bar and I'd just play my guitar and write.'

'You'd be near Granny, working, playing your guitar and writing. Sounds like the life of an artist.'

'Exactly! That's why they laugh.'

'Living life as an artist is laughable.'

That wide grin beams across his face again. 'Well, I know it's kinda… you know, romantic, I think they think I'm naive.'

'The image you have of what your life might look like feels romantic and maybe naive.' I suddenly become aware that I have no idea what this guy is studying. 'What is it that you study, Felix?' He looks a little startled and I feel like a parent bringing a child down to earth.

'Engineering. I'm studying engineering.' I feel myself speechless, surprised and want to smile but don't want him to feel laughed at.

'I notice that I feel really surprised by that. I thought you were going to say literature or music or something.'

'I know, I know.' He sits nodding, fiddling with a hole in his jumper.

'I don't know anything about engineering but I imagine it is also very creative.' I'm hesitant and don't know why I say this. I think I'm trying to be supportive.

'Yeah, it is, and I enjoy it, but I wanted to study literature.'

'What stopped you?'

'My parents felt it was important that I studied something I could do as a job.'

'They were thinking of your future in a different way to you.'

'Yeah, work has been so important to them, I guess they want that for me.'

'You have a different vision.'

'I think I have time to try a few things first.'

'And living in Paris, near Granny whom you love and has been poorly, working and playing your guitar and writing is a way of trying something different for a while.'

'Yeah, I think my parents worry I might just bum around, but I write a lot and I just, I just wanna try it.'

'So what's stopping you?'

'What?'

'What's stopping you trying it?'

'What, you mean now?' I nod. 'Well, I'm just finishing my degree, I've got to get my dissertation done, it's a lot of work and well I can't just stop.'

'You can't just stop. Because?'

'Because I've worked so hard and I'm nearly there.'

'It's been hard work and you're nearly there.'

'Yes.' We sit for a few moments with the sight of the end post hanging in the air. His eyes fill as he looks back at me. 'I think I just have to hold on.'

'I notice how your eyes have filled and the energy has dropped as you say that.'

'I know, it's a constant rollercoaster; I want to get off and stay on all at the same time. It's so tiring.'

'The rollercoaster is tiring for you, Felix.'

'Yeah, and then I feel all anxious again.'

'The rollercoaster and feeling tired brings about anxiety for you.'

'It's like, can I get it done, can I hold on?'

'Holding on and questioning your stamina is part of the anxiety?'

'Hmmm, yeah.' We sit for a few moments and I'm aware how I want him to jump on Eurostar right now with his guitar and notebook, back to Granny and her baking.

'I'm curious, Felix, that in an ideal world, if I had a magic wand and you could do anything you wanted right now – what would it be? Or what would you tell a friend in the same boat as you?'

Without hesitation he replies, 'I'd say just finish up, man, take a gap year in Paris, work and play guitar and then look to do the next thing – a Masters or whatever then.'

'Complete your study here, go to Paris and take things from there.'

'Sounds sensible, huh.' His head lowers.

'Sounds like a sensible plan for you. I noticed as you said that your head dropped down and you sounded critical and deflated.'

'My parents are sensible. I don't want to be sensible… I want… I want…' his eyes glaze again, 'I just want…'

'What? What is it that you want, Felix?'

'Live, I want to live you know to feeeeel alive.'

'You don't feel so alive.'

'I feel stuck and sensible.'

'Stuck and sensible and that doesn't feel like being alive.'

'I think I've had it too easy.'

'What d'you mean too easy?'

'My parents are very well off, they've paid for everything, they didn't want me to work while I studied and I've lived all over the world, but I… I… I just wanna make it on my own.'

'You feel it's all been too easy and you want to show you can do it on your own. Have you talked to your parents about this?'

'I try but I worry they feel I'm ungrateful.'

'So what are your options, Felix?'

'What d'you mean?'

'What options do you have to make it on your own, to feel unstuck, not sensible and alive?'

After a moment or two he replies, 'I can leave now and go to be with my granny. Or I can stay and finish the year and then go. But it's all so hard.'

'What's hard?'

'What if I decide to go now and it's a mistake?'

'Why don't you try and answer that? What if you leave now and it turns out to be a mistake?'

'Then I'd lose everything.'

'Like what?'

'My course, I won't have finished. It would've been a waste.'

'Anything else?'

'My parents would be right.'

'It would've been a waste and your parents would be proved right.'

'Yeah, but it might work.'

'What would that picture look like – if it was working?'

'I'd be happy. It'd be hard, but I'd be happy doing what I wanted to do, me choosing, working, playing. Might even find a girlfriend to play guitar with and write poetry for.'

He smiles at me and there is that glint like a flirtation, that energy in his eyes again.

'It'd be hard but you'd be happy and might find a girl to share your art with.'

'Yes! Exactly like that. I know, I know...' He shakes his head and I have no idea what's coming next. 'It's romantic, it's stupid, I know, I know.'

'Wow, Felix, that critical voice came in really fast, almost before you'd even had a chance to enjoy the scene you had created for yourself.'

'Fuck it, I know, I know *aarrggh!*' Tears form in his eyes and they look like frustration, maybe even a hint of rage.

'Whose critical voice is that, Felix?'

'Mine, err... no, my mum's. I can hear her, that's what she does with my dad, she criticises him when he gets his guitar out. He drinks a lot, my dad.'

'Why d'you think he does that?'

'To get away from her, he can just go into himself. When he plays guitar he's so lost in it, he's good too. He taught me how to play.'

'Dad taught you how to play.' He nods and a beam crosses his face as though he can hear music.

'Felix, I am curious to know if you imagine you would get the same response from both your mum and dad if you chose to leave university early?'

'I think he would go along with what she says but would secretly be glad for me. He kinda winks at me every now and then, you know.'

'What d'you take the wink to mean?'

'That he approves, that he likes what I'm doing, that he wants me to break free.'

'And how do you feel when you've seen the wink?'

'I feel really happy inside.'

I feel myself smile and I feel warm and happy inside too. I notice the time, draw our session to an end and make the next appointment. I walk around the room and stretch a little, then straighten the cushions and get a fresh glass of water ready for Fiona to arrive. I find myself fighting a wish to drift into my own world; a need to wallow. Half an hour into the session time I accept that Fiona isn't coming. I feel irritated. I could've wallowed for a bit longer and still had time to bring myself back for the new couple starting after Fiona's session. I check my phone and see the message. "Sorry for short notice, can't make it today, see you next week, will transfer fee, best wishes Fiona." It is coherent, considered, punctuated, and not the usual essay about how low she is feeling etc. Something feels changed.

Jack and Christine

I NOTICE THAT THERE SEEMS TO BE A FOG BEHIND my eyes. I have just written down the new clients' contact details like a dental receptionist. There is no air coming through the gaping window and the ambulance siren screams in to remind me that I would prefer a different setting for my therapy work, yet never find myself looking for one. I hear myself *tut* a sigh as I drop the notepad on the table. Looking up at the couple seated at each end of the sofa I address them:

'So that's the admin done. Maybe you'd like to begin by saying something about what brings you here?'

They look at me blankly. Then they look at each other blankly.

'Well, maybe you could ask us some questions to get us started,' states Jack.

'Like what?' I ask, feeling a little irritated as I thought I had, in fact, just asked a question.

He swallows looking rather perturbed. Christine sits looking down at her clasped hands. Unmoved, she's not going to talk so he answers for them both, 'Well... erm... I notice you didn't ask us how long we've been together.'

'I see. You would like me to ask you how long you've been together?' I look at him, then at her, then back at him. Another ambulance screeches by and I look between their heads and out of the window. I notice I really don't care how long they have been together and am a little startled by my feeling this way.

Jack responds, 'It seems like a reasonable question.'

'Why?' I ask. Quickly Jack turns his head and with a quizzical look seeks confirmation from his wife that what he is about to say is OK. He almost smirks as if to insinuate that I am stupid or something.

He looks back at me. 'Erm, because it might be relevant.'

'You think it's relevant.'

'Well I wouldn't be mentioning it if it wasn't.'

'OK, so the length of time you have been together is important to you. I hear that.'

'Yes, it is.'

'OK.'

'You still haven't asked how long it is.'

'I guess it's not so important to me. What I really hear is how important it is to you. Christine, you haven't spoken. Is it important to you too?' The air around us is tetchy causing eyes to widen as we all wait for something.

Christine shrugs her shoulders and lifts her eyebrows as the corners of her mouth simultaneously arc downwards. She sighs, 'We've been together a long time. Twenty-four years.'

'What does it mean to you to have been together for nearly quarter of a century?'

'It sounds like a long time when you put it like that,' says Christine with a more perked-up tone. She sits more upright now and appears to be interested in being here. Jack looks at his wife with his bottom lip slightly jutting out, like it has a life of its own. He looks stunned and furious. Without turning to look at her husband she continues looking at me, as if in defiance, knowing that he is still looking at her, as she speaks. 'Well you know, when you've been together a long time, things change.'

'What is it that you feel has changed and do you both feel this way?' I ask glancing at the couple equally.

'Hold on, hold on...' He waves his hands in the air, between the three of us, gesturing like a circus master holding the order of play in his hands and directing.

'Hold what?' I ask.

'Just hold on a minute.' He turns to his wife and swivels his torso, jacket twisting in the process. I'm thinking how creased that is going to be and wonder why he is wearing a woollen jacket in this heat. He shuffles and pulls the caught corner out hard as he looks at Christine. 'You've just jumped right in, there's other stuff.'

Christine sits up even more as she turns her head sharply to look at him sitting in the opposite corner of the sofa. She leans back slightly, looking affronted, with her pleated chin down and tucked under in contempt. Then she just turns back again and looks down at her fingers.

I intervene. 'I'm confused. Jack, you wanted me to ask how long you have been together, it seemed really important to you. Christine has stated how long you have been together and now we are exploring that. You don't wish to do that?'

'No. Well, yes, but – hang on...' He shuffles his backside forwards to the edge of the furniture and turns to look backwards at Christine. 'I don't want us to just jump in too fast.'

Christine raises her arm, looks at me and waves a hand, to prepare me to hear what is coming next. 'You wanted this Jack, you did, so now's your chance. This is what we are here for, there you go, tell her.' Her arm outstretched, hand open and still, as though offering up her husband for sacrifice. He watches with lips mouthing unformed words whilst no sound emerges. His wife just stares at him. No one says anything and I haven't the patience for games and long silences today. I wait as long as I can whilst the couple stare at one another.

'Neither of you have actually stated why you are here. All we seem to know so far is that it has something to do with the length of time you have been together and that things change.' I look at them back and forth, face goading a response.

Jack obliges. 'Yes, we know that, but before we get right into it there's a lot of stuff to look at, like – what's got us here.' He's looking really hot in that jacket.

'Well, it's up to you but we can also just get straight to the point of what was the final straw that made you choose this Friday. Why now?'

Christine jumps straight in.

'He's shagged about for years.'

'What?' he asks in disbelief.

'You have, that's why we are here now.'

'No!'

'No, you haven't shagged about?' Her face looks incredulous.

He looks back at her with facial muscles pleading, and that bottom lip looking to launch – something. Eyes wide and fixed. She stares back at him, quite pleased with herself I think.

'That's not what I meant. There's a lot…' He disintegrates back into the sofa and looks at me half caught out and half trying to stifle a grin. Then with irritation, 'I think there's a lot to talk about before we get to that'.

'Why?' demands Christine.

'What do you mean?' he asks.

'Why do we have to talk about a lot before we get to that?' She looks at me as though I should understand the statement and have an affinity with it. Is she wanting me to support her question? 'He keeps denying things.' I keep a blank face.

'I haven't denied anything… it's not… I haven't…'

'No, you deny it's significant.'

He looks at me some more, with his pleading face.

We sit in silence for a minute and I watch Christine bristle up her shoulders. Here it comes.

'He shags about, always has done. I haven't really minded, not once I got past the first time. Jo, was that her name?' She swiftly turns to look him in the eye, daring him to deny it. Sometimes couples use the space to shame each other. He's laid back on the ropes now, sweat down his face. Gravity pulling his arms to the floor. The weight of his gloves too heavy to lift. Can he make it back into the ring?

Too late, she's going back in for another swing.

'This one looks like she's here to stay though. Not going away so easy, is she Jack? Wants you to leave the wife and kids, does she?' Christine almost smirks through her tears of power and pain that smart.

'The kids are grown up,' he responds quietly.

'Yes, they are, so what's stopping you then?'

'What?'

'If it's not the kids, what's stopping you? Just leave.'

After a moment of looking at his hands whilst his thoughts catch up with his ears. 'You always knew?'

'Started with suspicion but then I dug a bit and now I always know the signs.'

'What signs?' Unconvinced of his own lack.

'Best suit, best underwear, train tickets in pockets, secret phoning, guilty looks, colleagues phoning thinking you were at home with me, slight changes in sex positions… loads of stuff, I just know.'

'Women fuck about too,' he says quietly.

She looks furious and turns all but purple. 'Oh, it's a gender war now, is it?'

'No, it's not a… what?'

'What do you want, Jack? I know this one is different so if you wanna go, go. Fuck off and go.' Her eyes are streaming a dare.

'It's not that simple, Chrissie.'

'It's that simple, Jack.'

'Well do you want me to go?'

'Don't you dare put this back on me. If I'd wanted you gone, I would've confronted you about the women you were shagging around with long ago.'

'Didn't it bother you? I mean it must say something about us if it didn't bother you.'

'Wasn't bothered! I was bothered alright, I was fucking devastated the first time. When I went to my sister's because she was suicidal – you remember? I missed Abby's twelfth birthday.' She directs her eyes to me. 'Abby is our eldest, she is twenty-two now.' She looks back at him. 'Well Kim wasn't suicidal, I was.'

'What? You made all that up, that stuff about the guy… you said she was being stalked or something… you lied about that?'

'So shoot me or divorce me – whatever. I decided there and then that week in Gloucester that I liked my life with you and the kids and accepted that, for some reason, you needed to do what you did to share little bits of yourself, that somehow, I didn't connect with… or something… I dunno. Maybe you were always just too immature to know and accept that one person can't be everything regardless of the stupid songs. I was happy and could live with it, besides I had the kids and the house, and—'

He interrupts. 'Oh, the kids – your life revolved around the kids and the bloody house.'

I watch the drama play out as things that need to be said are said.

'Yeah well, we've got – WE HAVE GOT – three great, emotionally stable kids so I am quite glad my life revolved around being a mother.'

'I'm a good dad!'

'Yes, you are Jack, you are, no one is disputing that and I will fight anyone who says otherwise, but if you don't want to be with me then just go – go.'

He sits there with eyes welling as they stare at each other. Christine fights hard to keep her emotions from overwhelming her stride.

He looks at me. Shakes his head at me. 'This was too fast. You did this too fast.'

'What is it that you think I've done, Jack?'

'You could've asked us some questions and led us in to this slowly so that it was more manageable.'

'You have assigned me the role of manager and pacer, Jack? It seems that you came to therapy today because you have reached a crucial point in your relationship and your lives. Well, that point just erupted.'

'I wasn't ready,' he says solemnly.

'Somewhere Jack, I think you were ready – you were the one who arranged this, you agreed with Chrissie earlier that this was your idea.'

'I know, I know, I just wanted it to be more… slower… I dunno… I don't want an explosion.'

'Life is explosive sometimes.' I hear myself say, *what?!*

He looks startled and this time his bottom lip juts out with pure indignance. 'I'm not sure this is how therapy should happen.'

'How should it happen?'

'Well... take our time, for one thing.'

'What is it you want to take your time to do, Jack?'

'What?'

'Look, you are both here because whatever it is that you want to say can't be said at home without some kind of mediator. Well go ahead – say what's got to be said.'

Surrender fills Jack's eyes and he turns to his wife.

'I don't know what I want.'

'Fuck off, Jack. If you think I'm waiting around while you decide you can think again. I have a life too; I'm disappointed sometimes too, and hurt and bored but this is what life is. You want life somewhere else then fucking go. You are released from mummy's apron strings – I should've cut them sooner. You brought me here to put me through stuff so you can work out what to do. Well live and die by your own sword, Jack, I'm done.' Christine stands up, looks at me, then back at him. 'Don't come home. I'll pack your stuff and deliver it to Graham's – she doesn't live far from there, eh – Carol is it – does she have kids too?'

She looks at me again, says thanks and leaves. He just sits there. Then he looks at the clock, then back at me. 'Now what?' he asks.

'I don't know, Jack.' Unexpectedly he jumps to his feet and I feel my heart quicken.

'I'm going to report you.'

'Yes, I think you should.'

'What?' He takes his wallet out of his back pocket, sifts through some notes and throws the money on the table.

'I feel like a prostitute,' I say, looking up at him from my seat. With ashen face and jutting lip, he turns on his heels and leaves.

Supervision

My supervisor, Roberta – Bob for short – is a tall, red-haired willowy woman with a very deep and commanding tone to her voice. We've worked together for ten years now. Like all relationships, we've had our ups and downs and don't always agree but our candour seems mostly productive. Supervision is mandatory for all counsellors and psychotherapists, is collegial and not hierarchical.

'Thanks for seeing me at such short notice, Bob, I do really appreciate it.'

'Not a problem, I'm glad we could meet up. You sounded somewhat panicked on the phone.'

'Hmm. I don't feel panicked but I do want to make sure that I'm handling my situation the best I can so that the client work is being held too.'

'OK.' Bob sits with her pen poised over her very large notebook, which has always puzzled me, though I've never raised my puzzlement.

'I've cancelled all client work for next week and then I'm on leave for a week anyway.'

'I see; it's unlike you to do this and so I'm wondering what prompted that action and also – are you alright?' I feel my eyes start to fill up, and as I begin to speak my mouth quivers. Looking at Bob, I raise my hand and gesture towards my own face as if asking for a moment's pause.

'You can see, I'm upset.' I manage some words.

'Yes, I can. How can I help?'

'Well you can't help with the tears, but I just want to check out that my client work is held. That I'm thinking straight where they're concerned.'

'OK, you say you have cancelled your client work. How did your clients take the news?'

'They were fine, except for Fiona because it means that I won't have seen her since she attended her ex-husband's funeral.' Bob flicks through her notebook and finds what has been discussed about Fiona before.

'Ahh, right here she is. Mmmm, was doing much better then ex-husband died and threw her into a complex grief process... identity who is she now... who will look after her now... still small in the seat... dad left... alright, what is it about Fiona that concerns you more than your other clients?'

'She's really hurting. Her grief has knocked her for six. The death of her ex-husband has triggered other stuff about her identity etc. I'm just concerned that if she becomes too low, and my taking a break is too impactful, then the steady improvement in her mood which she was experiencing will just drop and she may feel unsupported and vulnerable.'

'What was her reaction when you told her – you said all were fine except for Fiona – did you get to speak to her?'

'Yes.' I look to the corner of the ceiling to remember Fiona's response clearly. 'Actually, when I think of it she seemed alright. She never mentioned the funeral, although I didn't ask as I didn't want to open anything up on the phone. She thanked me for letting her know, hoped I was OK... and... erm... oh yes, she said she had a meeting with HR next week about when she might be going back to work. Funny, I'd forgotten that bit until just now.'

Bob smiles. 'You had forgotten she told you about her meeting?'

'Yes. Oh. She sounds like she's alright. I sometimes forget that clients get on with their lives in between sessions and that therapy is just fifty minutes out of a whole week's worth of living!'

'It can feel like it's their whole life sometimes in the intensity of a session.'

'Yes, it can. OK, so I feel better about Fiona.'

'So, you did—'

I interrupt. 'I also told Fiona about the first response emergency telephone number if there was a crisis and she told me once that she had considered calling the Samaritans – before we worked together, so... she's aware there is help if she needs it – though she said she won't need it. Sorry I interrupted you, Bob.'

'It sounds like you have attended to all the practicalities and signposted other options if a crisis occurs.'

'Yes, I did. It's OK, isn't it, you're right, *ahh*.' I collapse back into the seat with a long exhale and take a sip of water from the glass placed beside me.

Bob scribbles something in her book and then looks up and smiles at me.

'So. All practicalities attended to. What I noticed was that you had held on to details about Fiona that you didn't seem to hold on to about other clients.'

'Did I?'

'You said…' she looks at her notes, 'you mentioned the funeral when in fact she didn't, and you said she is really hurting, her grief has knocked her for six and seems to have triggered other stuff about her identity etc, but in fact when you spoke to her she seemed alright and told you about going to work for a meeting. I'm curious about the details you chose to bring here today.'

I sit for a moment or two, staring out of the window into the sunshine thinking of you and wondering where you are, what you're doing and if you have forgotten me.

'You seem to be working really hard to try and hold back tears.' My tears slip away and for a moment I cannot speak. Bob sits in wait, watching. I just keep staring at the geraniums in the window box peeping over and, eventually, bring my focus back into the room.

I fold the tissue between my fingers and look at Bob. 'My relationship has ended, I was alright, sad of course, but alright, and then suddenly it felt overwhelming – grief that is.'

'I'm so sorry to hear that. I didn't know that you were in a relationship but I'm very sorry to see you so sad about its ending.' We sit in a pause of silence as I mop up. Looking up from under my tissue. 'Thank you.'

Bob neither smiles nor grimaces but slightly nods her head.

'I saw a new couple, Jack and Chrissie. I'm not sure that I handled it well, it was a bit explosive in the end.'

'Explosive in what way?'

'Well, he had insisted they come to therapy, mainly on the pretence that they look at their twenty-four years of marriage. He is having an affair, has had many she said, and I think wanted it out in the open so that he could leave – though not sure about that. She'd known all along and called him out on it and so it all escalated a little faster than he would've liked. He blamed me, mainly because I just sat back and let it happen. He was angry. Then at the end I told him I felt like a prostitute.'

Bob couldn't stop her eyes from widening. 'How did it get to that point?'

'Well, actually I was a little irritated by them to be honest, so just gave space to let the drama play out. He criticised me for not taking things more slowly, but it was their pace and I left them to it. I was not going to be dragged into his game.'

'He was playing a game?'

'Yes, you know, he had an agenda, she was supposed to come along and fall into his trap so that he could leave and get her to take the blame, or some of it, or something, I don't know. I just felt used. We were at the end of the session, I was still sitting, he had stood up and all but threw the fee down on the table and I looked up at him and heard myself say "I feel like a prostitute"; he went white and left. I think he said something about reporting me.'

'"Prostitute" is a strong word and evokes a particular sentiment. You say you felt used.'

'Yes, like he was intending to use me and my work to manipulate his wife into taking the blame for him wanting to leave the marriage for this other woman. Like a cop-out, you know? Where's his responsibility?'

'I'm curious how he communicated that to you.'

'What, communicated what?'

'That he wanted to manipulate his wife into taking the blame so that he could leave. How did he communicate that he wanted to leave exactly?'

'Well he, he...' I sat for a moment. 'Oh. I don't think he did articulate it. Actually, she was the one who mentioned him leaving. It was more the way the session played out.'

'What d'you mean? Say more about how it played out.'

'He wanted me to ask questions to get them started, but I wasn't going to play into that, and then she just came out with the fact that he was having an affair and that she knew all along, and that she will pack his stuff up and he could go.'

Bob winces.

'Sounds a bit like a runaway train.'

'It was in a way. But look how she handled it. She knew what she wanted and handled it. She had known all along and was not going to sit around waiting for him to make the decision. She made it. She chose for her own life.'

'And he was angry with you.'

'Yes.' I stop for a moment and go back to looking out of the window. 'I know I could've perhaps slowed things down a little, though I'm not sure what the benefit would've been. We know that some couples use therapy to reveal something they can't approach at home. I don't know how he imagined her to react but he seemed shocked, speechless at what she did say and do.'

'How d'you feel about him?'

'What d'you mean?'

'Well, I've heard you say that she knew what she wanted and that she handled it; wasn't going to sit around and wait for a decision, and you are here asking where his responsibility was. What I hear in that, and please correct me if I'm wrong, but what I hear is you enjoyed her power over the situation, she took control. You enjoyed that about her, and that it shocked him.'

'I'm not sure I enjoyed his shock, but maybe I did. Yes, you're right, I did enjoy her power and decisiveness. She was also very upset but was refusing to show any sense of brokenness.'

'Brokenness, what do you mean by that?'

'Well, there he is "shagging about" – that's her term, not mine – she knew all along and now he creates this drama of coming to therapy and she's like "just fuck off and go" –

her words not mine. She wasn't broken, is powerful and is going to survive.'

'I see, you enjoyed her decisiveness, power and ability to survive.'

'Yes, I did to be honest, I did. As you are well aware, we find out who we are in these kind of painful events – how we manage the push and the pull.'

'Where was the pain in all this?'

'She cried, the whole time, but she maintained her poise and determination anyway.'

'And Jack? Where was Jack's pain?'

Doof. I suddenly feel stunned, blank, unable to access my thoughts or words. I can feel my cheeks get slightly warm and involuntarily swallow down a small glob of guilt.

'He cried too. Shit. I didn't attend to his pain, did I?'

'Well, maybe you did, maybe you didn't, maybe he wouldn't let you.'

'No, I wouldn't let me.' My eyes widen and I feel frustrated with myself. 'I couldn't see his pain. I so wanted her to show that she had power and could withstand, that I missed his pain… hmm that sounds like Meg and her mother… anyway, when I picture them now at opposite ends of the sofa, I saw him squirming, struggling with his jacket caught in the corner of the seat. He was hot and nervous, his bottom lip jutting out, maybe he was even bewildered. Shit.'

'I'm wondering if now I can go back to the point I made earlier about you holding on to parts of Fiona's experience where you remembered the funeral and complex grief, when in fact she had not mentioned the funeral at all when you spoke to her.'

'You think they are linked?'

'I have no idea, but you have brought them both here today, along with your own upset around your relationship ending.' I look at the ground between us and nod.

'Yes, they are linked, of course, all of it is linked. Fiona has been on my mind and I was looking forward to hearing and exploring how the funeral went for her. But she cancelled that session. In my mind it felt like it could be an important transition, after all there is no way back after death, and in a way, I wondered if it could even free her. I've been experiencing grief around the end of my own relationship and am nowhere near the point of feeling free from it yet, and by the time Jack and Chrissie came to me I think I was feeling angry.'

'Your own process of grief also played out in the session.'

'Yes, yes I see that.'

'We can't escape it, everything is always being played out one way or another to some extent. Do you think Jack and Chrissie will come back?'

'I have no idea, I mean in a way he got what he wanted in that it all came out into the open. What happened after the session I don't know. He may not trust me again, or he may decide he wants to come and have a battle. Who knows? No other appointments have been booked and I am on leave now.'

'How d'you think you will handle it if they come back?'

'Well, it depends what they lead with and what their situation is if they do come back, and I still trust that clients choose what to say and when. I could choose a little more mindfully my own responses though.'

'Which you usually do, so I don't want you beating yourself up too much about this. I also heard that Chrissie knew her own mind and had actually made her mind up long before the session even took place too. In a way, you were also kind of highjacked – or what was it you said "used"?'

'Haha, yes, indeed.'

'I don't wish us to drift into therapy, but as we have been alert to how your own relationship ending has impacted this session, I'm wondering if "feeling used" is in the mix somehow?'

I wait for an answer to arrive in my mouth. 'Yes. I felt suddenly used and discarded. It felt ludicrous and cruel that it could all end the way it did.' I stare back out at the geraniums thinking that Bob will take this to her supervisor of supervision – a never-ending cycle of reflection in the field of therapy. I think of an old friend who dislikes geraniums intensely. She says they are "old people's plants". I've always loved them. I must call my mother. I must call my friend Samantha too. I'm aware that I've now emotionally left the session, am exhausted and want to go home.

'Ahh, I see. Well, you see all that, and you are astute enough to be able to work it through now, I am sure. Are you back in therapy?'

'No, but I'm planning on checking back in. Plus, the main reason I'm taking this time off is to process my grief so that there is less chance of it getting muddled up in the client work – again!'

'Are you going away?'

'No, just pottering and walking locally.'

'Well, enjoy.'

Meg

'I'VE BEEN THINKING A LOT ABOUT MY DIVORCE and it was the darkest time but somehow I knew I was walking through the light. Often I'd get up about four o'clock in the morning, not having been to sleep, and walk for miles to try and tire myself enough to sleep. It cost me a lot to end the marriage, emotionally, but in a way I felt so alive – even if I was frightened most of the time.'

'It cost you and you felt frightened.'

'But when I walked before anyone was up, except the birds, I also felt energised and I'd make loads of plans.'

'Energetic planning.'

'Yeah. Stupid really.'

'It felt stupid.'

'The plans were mad.'

'You made mad plans.'

'Like, I wanted to go and live in Canada. I don't know why Canada, I've never been. But I see all those wide expansive pictures of mountains and trees and wooden houses and I felt such an urge to go.'

'What stopped you?'

'I had two children to bring up. I had to make everything stable again for them. I dunno, maybe I was a coward too – I mean what would I have done – how does it happen exactly when you hear of people just packing up and fucking off?'

'When you left your marriage, you imagined yourself in Canada but it felt in conflict with bringing up the children, and also maybe you felt cowardly by not going.'

'Maybe coward is a bit harsh, I did have the kids.'

'You both had the kids.'

'I know, I know, but I couldn't drag them away from Richard, I just couldn't. They'd been through enough upheaval.'

'And now?'

'What d'you mean?'

'I'm curious that at that time of rupture you found yourself contemplating… what was it you said… "fucking off", but you couldn't because of the children. Now you find yourself going over old ground about when your marriage ended and I find myself curious about what this recent ending means for you now that the children are grown.'

'I see. Well, I'm nearly sixty, where is there for me to go?'

'You don't think you have anywhere to go?'

'I retire in five years. I have to wait it out.'

'You have to wait.'

'Plus, I have the grandchildren, I don't want to miss out on them.' She seems to drift off somewhere; a dreamy translucence in her face. She smiles and looks up at me. 'I suppose I could go to Canada for a holiday.'

'Canada for a holiday.'

'Yeah. Teaching doesn't start until October; I could go for a month.'

'A long holiday.'

'I've often wondered what I may've missed out on.'

'You might've missed out.'

'If I'd gone to Canada when the kids were young – I could've, there were jobs you see – what would life have been like? Everything would have been different and me, I'd have been anonymous.'

'You would've been anonymous and everything would've been different to the life you've had since being divorced.'

'Oh, I dunno, that would've had its difficulties I guess. No matter where I was it was going to be difficult.' Her eyes, tear up. 'I just wish he hadn't ended it. Everything was alright.'

'Everything was alright as it was.'

'Now I've been thrown into having to create something new again, and I don't want to have to, I don't.'

'Change has been forced upon you.'

'I suppose something had to give in the end.'

'If you'd stayed together, how do you imagine the relationship playing out?'

'Well, she'd have died and we could be together.'

'In order for you and Len to be together, his wife would've had to die.'

'Sounds bad.'

'Sounds drastic.'

'How else was it going to happen?'

'I'm guessing there are lots of choice points before we get to the stage someone has to die for us to live our life as we wish.'

'Yes but, he couldn't leave, I didn't want him to leave.'

'Why didn't you want him to leave?'

'I've thought a lot about the unavailability of Len – the idea of unavailability you harp on about, you know? I think it's important to me, I need it.'

'You need unavailability.'

'Yeah. I need something to want, something to long for.'

'Longing is important to you.'

'It's important to everyone but we forget.'

'Who forgets?'

'Everyone. When we think we have something, we close our hand around it and squeeze it to death.'

'The life gets squeezed out of it.'

'That's what happened in my marriage. It was nobody's fault. But we thought we were safe, secure and that was a mistake. We forgot that we needed to keep longing.'

My chest feels squeezed. 'Isn't longing painful?'

'Yes!' She sits up straight in her seat and all but lurches herself forwards. 'Yes! That's the point, we must feel the pain. I need to feel the pain, the ache, oh my God the ache.' Water fills her eyes and yet I see a fire lit behind them.

'Aching with pain feels necessary for you.'

She stares at me and then brings her hands up to her face and releases deep-throated sobs into her palms. I want her to fall, to curl up, thrash about, let the sobs rip through her. But no. She comes to stillness.

'I won't be caged.'

'I'm not sure I know what you mean.'

'I won't be caged by grief, or love.'

'Grief and love won't cage you.'

'No. It must all just flow through me. Sounds grand, that's not what I mean.'

'You don't mean it to sound grand.'

'No. It hurts, fuck it hurts so much that sometimes I want to die. But I won't. I'm alive if it hurts. I won't be dead in the cage.'

'If you're hurting, you're alive.' She barely nods, 'Sounds masochistic.'

'No, that's just life.'

'I'm aware, and I realise it may sound trite, but I don't want you to hurt too much.'

Meg smiles. 'What's too much?'

'Hmmm… I guess I don't want you to go under.'

'We must! We must go under, don't you see? Otherwise there's no rise. And I will rise.'

'What's the rise for you?'

'That I keep longing.'

'For what, who?'

'Someone, no one, everyone, I don't know what I'm longing for, but that doesn't matter now. Now I have to change something.'

'Like what? What will you change?'

'Well, I shall resign from my job. I've stayed too long already.'

I feel myself wince and want to say "you're grieving, don't make any big decisions just yet". But I have to bite my tongue and I feel it almost blocking the back of my throat.

'You will resign from your job. Remind me, what is it you teach again?'

'I teach literature.'

I feel myself flood with warmth and try to hold back a smile that wants to dance upon my face singing "but of course, but of course". Literature knows how to long, to ache, to sing and dance.

'What will you do?'

'Don't know… live abroad for a while, that's if Europe will have me, though why would it? Or maybe I'll go further afield after all and try Canada.'

'What will you do there?'

'What all teachers of literature dream of – write.'

'You will write.'

'Yep. Write and long and long and write. I mean, really, what the fuck else is there?'

It's not a question she is wanting me to answer.

'I… I… was OK with the way things were.' Her head drops from the previous rise of anger.

'And yet that day you turned up at his house, suggests that there was part of you that wasn't OK with the way things were.'

'Well, no, I mean I was hurt, angry, I wanted… I dunno, I wanted…'

'You wanted.'

'I wanted us to be together – we had a chance if she knew.'

'If his wife knew about you, then you'd have had a chance to be together fully.'

'Yes.'

'That's where your imagination takes you – being together fully.' Meg stares.

'I kidded myself for twenty years. I thought that twenty years made it special, extraordinary but all the time I was secretly hoping h…e'd… le…ave.' She barely got the last two words out and I watch her body jolt up and down, up and down as she cries out that last sentence. We are always kidding ourselves about something.

'D'you think I should've told him that I wanted him to leave? You know instead of going along as though it was all fine?'

'I'm wondering how you would've been able to do that, given that you only just now seemed to realise it yourself? Only a moment ago you said how the longing and pain was important.'

'Well, I've only just said it out loud, but if I'm honest, there were lots of times that I knew I wanted him to leave and be with me.'

'What d'you feel stopped you from acting upon that knowing?'

'Oh I dunno. I just never want to be THAT woman.'

'You don't want to be THAT woman. Do you mean your mother or a kind of woman?'

'Both, I mean I can't bear those women who whine, become victims you know – take responsibility.'

'Like you did.'

'Yes. No. Oh I don't know, it's such a muddle.'

'You feel in a muddle.'

'I just, I didn't make demands, I agreed my place in this and I honestly, honestly thought I was OK in it. I could've found many ways to tell his wife many times, especially when I was feeling low on my birthday or Christmas or something, you know. But I didn't.'

'You came close.'

'Yes, I came close.'

I watch her as that sentence settles in the wince upon her face.

'In all honesty, part of me wishes she'd have seen me that day or that I'd lost the plot and just gone up to her and told her, see what the difference would be.'

'If you follow that wish where does your imagination take you?'

'That she'd have thrown him out.'

'And then what?'

'He'd have had to come to live with me.'

'He wouldn't have had any choice but to be with you.' My response smarted; I can see it on her face, eyes darting all around the room until they settle on her hands holding the tissue.'

'No, it's just all fantasy. I know deep down, I know, he didn't choose me.'

'You wanted to be chosen but weren't.'

'I think I was chosen, partly. For twenty years I was chosen. I guess I have to work out now where I go from here.'

'Where to go from here.'

'I don't want to be alone, but I'm in no hurry to get into another relationship. I mean that's the right thing to do, isn't it, not jump in?'

'I think whatever you choose is right for you.'

'Yes, but I mean you wouldn't advise me to go straight into another one would you?'

'That's not my call to make.'

'I know, but you know, what's the research? I mean, should I wait and feel better, or just jump in and, fuck it, you know? Do what I want?'

'Which part of what you just said is what you want?'

'Well I mean, I dunno, that's why I'm asking. Should I just say yes and go for it or work all this out first?'

'What are you working out?'

'The end, should I deal with that?'

'Should you deal with the ending of you and Len? What's attached to the "should"?'

'Well what's the best thing, will I get hurt again if I jump in too soon?'

'There's always a risk of getting hurt no matter when we jump in, that's the point.'

'But if I jump now, is there more of a risk of things not working out?'

'What would be working out?'

'That we would stay together, it wouldn't end.'

'Are you talking about someone in particular?'

'What?'

'When you speak I have a feeling there is a possibility of you jumping now with someone.'

'Hmmm... yeah. There's a guy at work I've known for a couple of years, we're really good friends. He's divorced but I've never told him about Len, I think I just somehow managed to convey I wasn't interested. Actually, I think I've had "fuck off" written across my forehead for twenty years without realising.'

'You feel you've been communicating "fuck off" to other potential relationships?'

'Yeah, stupid, given what's happened. But I guess I'm free now and could be more open to Pete.'

'You seem to be saying that you didn't make yourself free for other relationships whilst you were with Len.'

'I didn't. I was committed. How foolish of me.'

'Foolish sounds harsh.'

'Maybe, but I feel stupid. I feel like I've lost out on so many other possibilities.'

'You feel that you limited yourself somehow? Are you saying you wish you'd chosen differently?'

'Yes, of course, then I wouldn't be in this situation... I mean... you know... *hoh*... yes... I see... I know... I just had no eyes for anyone else when I was with Len... *hoh* stupid... she didn't either, did she?'

'His wife?'

'No, my mother.'

'I see.'

'That's what she did, didn't she; held on for dear life not daring to tread elsewhere. Well fuck that. I like Pete, we have a lot in common, in fact when I think about it I spent – spend – more time with him than Len anyway. What am I waiting around for?' A blankness remains in her face after she said that; there's no muscular expression as her eyes reveal a sharp glint of defiance. I notice I have a doubt about her wishes to not be waiting around.

'What are you waiting around for?'

'Dunno, I honestly just dunno.'

That is the final sentence of the session. We arrange for our next four sessions and I have a feeling that our work is coming to an end, for the moment at least. Grief is an oscillating beast, and I feel a little mistrust that Len has gone away for good.

Luke

I GO INTO RECEPTION TO HAVE A CUP OF TEA WITH Debbie, the receptionist, before Luke arrives. I notice that I'm enjoying the banter. I go back downstairs and get the room ready for Luke. At his allotted time, I go back to reception to collect him but he isn't there. I loiter for a while, feeling a little churn in my belly, aware that Luke is never late, ever, and he has always turned up to every session. I wonder if he may have felt abandoned when I took off, even though he sounded alright on the phone. Luke arrives within five minutes, apologising as he got stuck in traffic, leaving later than he should have. It is really unlike him and I notice how I like that. Something has changed. I watch him settle into his seat. He looks well, has lost some weight. We sit looking at one another for a few moments.

'A lot has happened whilst you've been away... or doing what you've been doing.' I ignore the inquisitive hint. 'Cherry and I are seeing a counsellor. Together.'

'Couples counselling. I see.'

'Yeah, she broke down one night. Said she had seen me with Rebecca in the car. I was a mess.'

'You were in a mess when Cherry revealed she had seen you.'

'Yeah. And yet I was also relieved. I know that probably sounds bad but it was out. She knew. It was really bad. We were up all night.'

'Sounds exhausting.'

'It was. As you'd cancelled our session I didn't want to ask you in case you were ill or something, so we found a counsellor together. A bloke so that's a bit different for me – you know, man to man.'

'It sounds healthy that you chose together. And a bloke, as you put it, no doubt changes the dynamic for you.'

'It really does, but I'm not sure how. I think Cherry feels safer. I watch her and she hangs on his every word, but he keeps pulling her up about it. It upset her to start with but now I can see her getting more confident.'

'It feels different having a male counsellor but you don't know how and you watch how he affects Cherry.'

'Yeah, I love it. She stands up more for herself. Her family are a bit shocked that she's not putting up with their shit anymore. She's got 'em all running around helping out instead of doing everything herself.'

'And you, what's it like for you that she is standing up for herself?'

'I like that too. It's mad I know but I feel freer somehow. I don't have to be the strong one all the time and because she is speaking her mind more we are doing more and making decisions about us. Not just that, because she is speaking up more I have to look at me.'

'Her speaking up makes you look at you.'

'Yeah. I could've done what he's been doing: helping her, listening to her instead of cheating on her. I feel scared that I could lose her, you know, I mean really lose her. I mean she is a fantastic person. I always knew that and now she is feeling it, she could leave me.'

'What's that thought like?'

'That hasn't changed. It would kill me if she left.'

'It would kill you.'

'Yeah. I've hurt her really badly but seeing her like this makes me scared she could just go, you know.'

'She could just go.'

'Yeah. The counsellor, the guy, the work is going really well. He slows everything down so we can see how we're reacting to each other, in the minute as it happens. It was really irritating at first, but it's really good now. We look forward to the session, like it's our night out.' Luke laughs a belly laugh.

'I don't think I've ever heard couples work be described like that before. I'm glad that it's working for you. For both of you. I think couples work is so valuable. I wish more people would engage with it.'

'I know. I mean I should've suggested that before, then maybe I wouldn't have got in such a mess.'

'You feel if you had gone to couples counselling earlier that you'd have avoided the mess somehow?'

'Well, I know hindsight is always easy. But for instance, learning what happens for Cherry when I get all excited and sit in front of the telly watching the match has been really important. I always thought she was just pissed off with me, naggy, and then I'd get all "I've been to work all week" *blah blah blah* – but no, it wasn't all about me. It was about all the crap she deals with all week with the kids and her mum and dad and stuff. Just hearing the football on the telly triggers this feeling for her that she says makes her just want to scream. He has said that maybe she should have some therapy just for her too. So… who knows.'

'It sounds like it's been revelatory for you; looking at how you respond to triggers and how that gets played out between you both.'

'Yeah, it's been really good.'

'Luke, I am really struck by what you said earlier, that Cherry could just go now.'

'Yeah.'

'Well, this might sound brutal, but Cherry could've always gone.' We sit momentarily letting the statement sink in and he drops his head, nodding as he does so.

'Yeah, you're right. You know, I wonder if I had the affair just to push things.'

'To push things. Can you say more?'

'Well, it's like being a kid again. I used to push my mum 'til I could get what I wanted. Cherry was busy and stressed and we argued, and I know Rebecca cared for me, and me her, but maybe I pushed everything to the limit.'

'You feel you pushed things to the limit, like you used to push your mum.'

'Yeah, not on purpose, but I can't really come up with a reason why I had an affair. Not really and it could've caused – well did cause in a way – so much damage.'

'And yet you described many reasons why you loved Rebecca in our previous sessions and how the relationship met a different part of you.'

'Yeah, yeah I know, I know. It did, but to be honest I think I was just escaping or maybe experimenting.'

'You were escaping or experimenting.'

'It was good to feel a different part of me but, to be honest, I always felt better with Cherry, I dunno, at home, even with all the crap of work and the house and kids and stuff. I felt at home. If Cherry wasn't Cherry, I'd be out on my ear.'

'So, in a way, your experiment has proved to you how much Cherry loves you.'

A blanket of silence drops from the ceiling and hovers about an inch from our heads. With startled eyes, Luke bursts into tears. A relentless, deep sobbing cuts through the silence and shatters it. Male sobs roar, with a deep and childlike screech that vibrates off the walls and bounce back into the room. Luke doesn't move. He just stays in his seat and lets it pour out. It feels harrowing and traumatic. I have to stay put in my seat and watch as it all vibrates through me, off me. I have to hold this space so that he can experience fully his pain, and so that he can heal it too. I am no healer, I am sure of that. I can only be the holder of his secrets and to give him the opportunity to move freely through his own experience for fifty minutes at a time. But here something seems to have happened, something experienced in a way that it hasn't been before.

I watch the path of sobbing, tears, snot and strewn tissues until, eventually, it subsides and the air quietens. The blanket of silence has lifted. It takes some time for Luke to settle himself. I can hear sirens and the traffic passing. I really must find a better space more conducive to this work, even if clients don't seem to notice the screeching sirens, I do, and they go through me whilst I am trying to be attentive and work with a client's distress.

'*Hoh*.' He breathes out deeply and softly. It is a fragile breath.

I stay still and offer my eyes as a welcome invitation to speak, keeping my mouth silent for as long as Luke needs it to be. He breathes in and out a few times more.

'*Hoh*, I don't know what happened, but that hurt like hell.'

'It hurt like hell.'

With mouth quivering, 'Yeah, like hell.'

I feel my own body begin to settle, shoulders relax, belly floods with a warmth and I take in my own deep breath.

'When you said that, about Cherry lovin' me,' his mouth quivers again upon saying the words, 'I saw my mum and Cherry like they blurred in a picture in front of me, and it all just exploded in my chest. Those words, you know... "I just wanted to know that I was loved"... I didn't know that's what I was doing.'

'You just wanted to know that you were loved.'

His mouth quivers again. 'Yeah. I mean I knew I was but I don't think I ever felt it in my body until just now... God... that was powerful.'

'It was a powerful feeling in your body, feeling loved.'

'Oh God, yeah. Yeah.' He sits nodding his head and exhaling, blowing out little breaths that seem to come from the deep.

'I'll be honest, I was coming here today to say I think we can stop, you know, 'cause of the couples' work going so well. I thought I didn't need this anymore. But maybe I do. I didn't expect this. Mind you, I've never really expected any of the outbursts. You're good, you're good at this.'

'Luke, you have come here week after week and done the work. I think you're good at this.'

We pencil in four sessions with a question mark by the fourth as a possible ending. An occasional sob-like breath escapes from Luke's mouth as he gathers himself to leave. He takes a sweet from the bowl on his way out. I smile inside, either he didn't realise he had taken it, or he did. Either way it is a significant step.

I wedge the door open for a while as I potter around the room, fluffing up cushions and cleaning water glasses. I open the window to let in the air and the sound of traffic. Noisy life passing by the window. It's a strange business being a therapist. I sit for a while scribbling in my notebook.

Rosie

ROSIE WALKS INTO THE ROOM AND TAKES HER SEAT less hesitantly than previous sessions. She smiles at me and reaches for the glass of water, though I feel she doesn't really want a drink.

'Well, I feel a lot better.'

'You do?'

'We've been away... me and Jerry; he booked us a long weekend in the lakes as a surprise.'

'How was that for you?'

'I'll be honest, I was irritated at first. I'm not very good with surprises and I had stuff to do, but the kids got involved and told me to forget everything and just go.'

'Surprises throw you into a state of irritation.'

'Well, I guess I like to know where I am and what I'm

doing, but they were right, everyone was right. We had a lovely time and talked a lot.'

'The trip gave you an opportunity to talk.'

'Yeah, after that big row we had, something's felt different between us anyway. I cried a lot the first night because we were up talking until about four in the morning. I dunno, too much wine maybe… or maybe we don't get too much time at home, which is mad 'cause the kids aren't there, but we still don't seem to have time together. And then with this…' she glances down at her right breast and shrugs her arm up '… anyway we found ourselves talking a lot.'

'You talked more and into the early hours.'

'Yeah. I didn't realise how frightened he'd been.'

'Jerry had been frightened.'

'Yes. And he didn't know what to do and he said I seemed to just carry on so he did too. He said he was really upset about Matt taking me to appointments and thought that maybe I'd leave him for Matt! Can you imagine?'

'Can I imagine? Can you imagine?'

'No! Absolutely not – most of time it was convenient for Matt to take me is all, Jerry was at work in London, but I can see how it all looked now and I felt really bad when Jerry was telling me on Friday night. He looked like he could've burst into tears. I felt awful and stupid…'

'You felt stupid.'

'Like, how did I not see? How could I not know what impact this all had on Jerry?'

'When you ask those questions, what answers do you come up with?'

'I think, as I've said before, I was just in it. It's weird but it's like it was mine, belonged to me even though I didn't ask for it or want it and I just locked myself into it 'cause I think I felt I had to get rid of it. I mean I know I didn't, the surgeon and oncologist did that but, you know, I was responsible for how I was going to respond.'

'Your response to the situation and treatment was your responsibility.'

'Yeah… but… I didn't choose my response really, it's not like I sat down and thought, *well this is how I'm gonna respond*, I just did what I did.'

'Would you do anything differently?'

'Maybe, talk to Jerry more, but I probably wouldn't. Being self-sufficient seems so engrained. No, it's not just that, it's how Jerry and I go on. I'm still me and still intact – apart from the ugly scars of course, but me and Jerry in the end, we do what we do and we always talk eventually. I think maybe I lost trust in that for a while.'

'You lost trust.'

'I think I felt really vulnerable and kinda shut down to deal with it. In the end, I was the one who had to deal with it and I think I was really scared about how Jerry would respond. I've watched Matt over the years come and go with women and I think somewhere, deep down, I was really scared Jerry wouldn't want me anymore.'

'You felt vulnerable and feared you would lose Jerry.'

'I think so, even though I know things are solid too but this, this throws you, and I was scared.'

'Although things felt solid you also felt scared and both you and Jerry feared that the other could leave.'

'I was really surprised because he said he knew; he knew that I was scared but that he also knew how I go inside myself and distance myself from him. He said he trusted that I would come back when ready.'

'How did you feel when he said that, Rosie?'

'I felt really secure and it made me cry a lot. Like I put myself through so much but he was there all along.'

'You feel secure knowing Jerry was there all along.' She smiles and nods a few times as she touches the cushion on the sofa by the side of her. 'We had sex for the first time in five months. I cried all the way through… and I think the wine helped me to be not so conscious of my scars. It was fine, not our usual… it felt… I dunno strange, new, like being nervous the first time.' She smiles and winces all at the same time.

'It felt strange and new, like having sex for the first time.'

'Yes, but also strange because we knew it wasn't the first time so it was also familiar, it was safe and kind, I dunno… I dunno what I'm talking about, I've been having sex with this man for nearly thirty years.'

'It feels different.'

'Everything feels different. I know I was wanting things to be different but I also want things to be the same.'

'Yes, you've spoken before about that tension of things being so changed and yet the same.'

'I'm guessing that's just life though, it changes constantly but we don't notice until something major like this happens, you know, something that threatens everything.'

'Everything felt threatened.'

'Yeah: my health, my marriage, seeing the kids grow up, get married and have families of their own. I had moments when everything flashed before me and I saw it all disappear.'

'You saw your life and future hopes disappear.'

'I did, but I couldn't look at that, I couldn't bear those feelings so I just kinda dug my heels in and got on with it.'

'The feelings were too much to bear so you got on with things the best you could.'

'Yes, I did – I did the best I could, I did.' Rosie smiles to herself again. 'And it's alright, isn't it, I mean it's gonna be alright too. I'm a boob down but I'm alright and everyone else is alright.'

'Everything is alright, Rosie.' We sit for what seems like an age in the noise of those four words.

'Jerry asked me what I wanted to do about work as I'm due back next month.'

'What was that like for you to be asked given the things you've said here about wanting something to change.'

She chuckles, which took me a bit by surprise. 'Oh, well, I did talk about the tea shop idea and he was really good and he listened and said we could look at all those options and he could do a business plan and stuff – that's what he does, you see, he's in business and accounting, but... well, I don't think I really want to up sticks and move up there, I mean it would be a completely different kind of life.'

'The difference feels too much.'

'It does, and the upheaval. I mean I've had enough of that this last four months or so. But we did talk about me going part-time because when I go back next month it will be a phased return but I can stay part-time if I want. I can see how the part-time goes and if I want to develop something as an independent celebrant I can. I got quite excited when Jerry and I talked about it and he's looking to drop a day too or at least have a day working from home once a week so that we can have more time together.'

'All sounds very productive and somehow, I don't know, a meeting point between you and Jerry and your desire for change.'

'Yeah, it felt good. It felt like it was when we were young when we used to plan. I think we just got stuck in the rhythm of life, kids and work, but I guess things can change if we want them to, even if bad things happen.' She glances down at the right breast again.

'Rosie, I notice you often glance down at your right breast when you mention change.' Her eyes fill up so quickly and large tears fall.

'It's a massive change – massive – and I still can't quite believe it… believe it's happened to me.'

'A massive change and it's happened to you.'

'I know it's random, I know, I know – and why not me, why not? But you know. The reality sometimes shocks me and I feel so sad.'

'It's random and shocking, and sad too, Rosie. And it happened to you – your shock, your sadness.' Rosie has a really good sob that seems to come up from deep within the belly. I sit still, watching her sobs and tears and then weirdly feel my right breast twitch, like a speedy shooting twinge. Maybe I need to check my own breasts when I get home. She blows her nose, wipes her face and takes a drink of water.

'It comes up like that occasionally, but that's OK, isn't it? I mean that's normal, it'll take time.'

'Normal or not, it's how it is for you, Rosie.'

'Yeah, and I'm OK in between, I mean I haven't gone under.'

'Gone under?'

'You know, stuck in bed, depressed, drinking, gone off the rails. I mean I'm OK.'

'You're OK.'

'We are mostly, aren't we?'

'Who?'

'People. I see a lot of people in all kinds of situations and it's amazing how we cope with what life throws at us.'

'I see, yes I agree. I think we are much stronger than we think when push comes to shove.' I notice how her narrative has gone out to the wider world.

'As long as we don't think about it too much and just get on with it.'

'Well, I think it's different for everyone.'

'Yeah, but we have to get on, don't we, in the end.' I smile and confirm neither one way nor the other as this feels like Rosie going back into her self-sufficiency mode. I wonder what it was in life which shaped that side of her.

'Part of your attitude to life is to get on with it.'

'Yeah, I mean we suffer, don't we? Life throws up such awful stuff sometimes but aren't we strong really… you know, we do get on, in the end, I know we have to make the effort but "no point dwelling", as my nan always said.'

'Nan said no point in dwelling.'

'Well, she was strong, I mean you couldn't argue with her, she'd just feed you until you got better if you were ill or else just say "pull your socks up and get on with it", different generation I guess.'

'Maybe not so different – I hear you say the same thing about getting on with it.'

'I know, I know but I did want to crumble at times.' Rosie shuffles in her seat, straightens her blouse and sits upright, poised.

'There were times when you wanted to crumble, Rosie.'

Her eyes have the faintest glaze. 'I did, I thought, *I'll just stay in bed under the duvet, I'll just stop.*'

'I'll just stop.'

'Just hand over.'

'Hand over.'

'Yeah, you know that "stop the world I want to get off" feeling?' I nod. 'It was all so relentless, I just wanted to sleep my way through it and have it over so I could wake up and then get back to life again.'

'There were times you wanted to be asleep for the gruelling process that you went through to become well again.' Rosie's tears become a little more formed.

'*Ah ha*, yep, just sleep through it and wake up and it'll all be over: the pain, the torment of questions, all that stuff we've talked about.'

'If you could have just slept through it all and not experienced the pain, torment and questions.'

'I know it's a stupid thing to say, I know, but what's all

the pain and torment for when you could just go to sleep, wake up and have not known?'

'Sounds like that's another way of asking something you thought about earlier – what does this experience give you?' We sit for a few moments as Rosie ponders, I assume on that last statement, but who knows.

'You're right, I keep coming back to the same thing: what has it given me? I want so much for it to have been meaningful.'

'What meaning could you give it, Rosie?'

'Bloody hell, none! It has no meaning; the cancer came and it went and what am I left with?'

'What are you left with?'

'A bloody ugly scar where my breast used to be and… and I dunno, Jerry and I might be closer, I might change work. I am looking at my life, but really what's changed? I mean really, what has changed? Nothing! In a way nothing has changed… except…'

'Except?'

'Except, I worry it might come back and I don't think I can go through it again.' Now the tears are full and on the move.

'You worry it may come back, Rosie.'

'I haven't said that out loud before. It's like I know now that my body is really capable of cancer. I've been really positive with everyone, but yes there is a nag that now I've had it once it could come back. I mean they've said there's no reason, but you can't help wonder.'

'It is a nag there in the background, like background noise to your life that wasn't there before.'

'Exactly like that yes… but… I come back to my nan, you gotta just get on, 'cause this is it – this is life for me now.'

We sit for a few moments in this statement and I notice that we have come to time. Rosie decides that this is our last session for now and that if anything bubbles for her again she might come back, though I suspect she won't. I suspect Rosie will get on.

Fiona

Later I sit in the therapy room with a concern in my belly that Fiona may not turn up but instead she arrives early, sitting in the waiting room, groomed, smiling and taking up some space. She walked through to the room with a slight spring in her step. As she sits down I notice that there was no pre-arrangement of the bin and box of tissues. She's also holding a coffee beaker.

'I'm sorry that I didn't turn up for our last one. I know it's been a long time now.' Fiona grins and I notice that I feel intrigued.

'I notice that you are grinning.'

'I'm back at work.' Swiftly said through a wide smile.

'I do remember you saying on the phone that you had an appointment with HR – so you went back to work? I notice that you look more upright and… I don't know, lighter somehow.'

'Well, after I last saw you, Jason's wife, Lesley, came to visit me. I think it was the same day actually. I was mortified because my house was a tip and I was just curled up on the sofa looking bedraggled. Anyway, she was so kind to me. She said that Jason really cared for me and always worried I was alright. She always knew about the cards and flowers. She said that it must've been really hard for me when he died and was concerned that I may be alone. She asked me to attend the funeral in the car with her and the boys. I did go to the funeral, but not in the same car in the end. I didn't feel it was quite right. But I did sit with the family during the service and Lesley and her family were very kind to me.' Fiona gently tears up but not enough to be in need of a tissue.

'Fiona, that seems like a momentous event in the midst of your grief. What a remarkable hand of friendship to be offered.'

'I know. I was shocked. Of all the people around me, Lesley was the one who made everything suddenly shift.'

'Everything suddenly shifted for you, Fiona.'

'Yes. Absolutely everything. Her kindness. She came in and made me a cup of tea. Me. She had just lost *her* husband but came in and made *me* a drink. And it was easy being with her. It's like we kind of knew something together – what we were both going through. We shared something.'

'You both knew and shared something that you were going through.'

'Yeah, and I realise as I just said that, that we shared Jason too. We both shared a part of his life and somehow, she is sharing him with me now. Like a future. Mad I know. The children are lovely and it's so hard for them but they are doing really well. The older one really looks like Jason. That's odd and was hard for me at first, it was like looking at Jason when we were young. And I thought that's what our children would've looked like. Though I always wanted a little girl.' She smiles with no hint of a tear or sadness.

'The sharing that you're experiencing from Lesley feels like a future.'

'Yes. I know it probably sounds weird but I feel like I have a future. Does it sound weird? My family think it's weird.'

'Your family think everything you do is weird.' We both laugh. 'I notice that I'm feeling pleased for you, Fiona. That amidst such shock and grief a friend has come forward for you and you seem to have lifted out of that very low mood.'

'I have, haven't I? Don't worry, I know it could come back.'

'You feel it could come back.'

'Well, why wouldn't it? I know that my depression, if that's what it was, wasn't all about Jason. I think I put all my focus on him.'

'Like he was a hook?'

'Yes! Exactly like that. He became the hook, well our marriage ending became the symbol for all that I was unhappy with.'

'A symbol for all that you were unhappy with. I am curious about *all* the unhappiness.'

'It hasn't all gone, don't worry. I know there is stuff about how I feel about myself, and especially my dad. While you've been away I've been thinking a lot. I watched Lesley be so brave and kind and keep herself going for her children. I really admire her and it made me remember that I used to be strong. Anyway, when I went to the HR meeting they offered me a phased-return so I took it. I go full-time again next week. People said they've noticed a difference and I went out with them last Friday after work for a drink.'

'What was that like for you, Fiona?'

'I was a bit scared, like I had a neon light over my head saying "watch out – depressive in the house".'

'You felt marked out somehow.'

'Not really, that was my fear, but that's not what it was like. It was lovely. I felt like an old me even though I'm not the same. Weird isn't it. That I know I've changed and yet somehow feel the same. I also think all the time I felt an outsider to the group that maybe I kept myself apart from them.'

'You kept yourself separate. What's it like having that feeling of change and sameness both at the same time?'

'It feels safe, familiar. Yes, I feel safe and familiar with myself.'

'Safe and familiar with yourself.'

'Yeah, I can trust myself – oh God – oh...' Tears fill her eyes and she reaches out from her seat to take a tissue from the box.

'That looks like it touched something really important for you.'

'I think I'd forgotten what it was like to trust myself. All my feelings got in such a muddle before.'

'Your feelings got muddled and so you lost trust in yourself.'

'I did. Things seem so much clearer now.'

'You have some clarity.'

'I loved Jason very much, I did, I still do somewhere but… this is going to sound bad… in a way I feel freer. It's like he had to die before I could be… I dunno… released or something. Does that sound bad?'

'It feels bad for you to say that?'

'I didn't wish him dead, but that he is, means I can't keep wondering what if, you know, keep wondering if things could be different. It's like the possibility has been taken away. It's not an option, if you know what I mean?'

'You no longer have to spend time asking what if and wondering about possibilities.'

'Yeah. I cry when something happens or I watch the news and I think Jason is not in the world to see that. It's really strange knowing someone is just gone – gone out of the world. But my crying feels alright. I don't sink into that hole, like before.'

'You can grieve and cry and carry on without sinking.' Fiona smiles, moves a cushion around on the sofa and looks around the room.

'I don't think I've really looked at the room before. I like that picture, is it yours?'

'No, it belongs to the centre.'

'Ahh, nice. I'm thinking of painting – the house – not making a picture.'

'Why not a picture?'

'Oh, dunno, don't think I could paint.'

'I imagine you could try anything you wanted to, Fiona.'

'Ahh thanks, who knows, eh?'

'Indeed, who knows.' We sit just looking at each other for a while and the silence feels empty somehow. 'I'm wondering Fiona, what this space is for you now as things seemed to have changed so much?'

'You mean therapy?'

'Yes.'

'I was thinking that on the way over. I don't want to give it up as I think there is still stuff that I need to look at. You know, how did I drop to my knees in the first place? I'd like to continue, if that's alright with you?'

'Of course, does this time and day suit on a regular basis?'

'Yeah, this is fine.'

'OK, let's book in the next six and see where we go from there.'

Felix

I NOTICE FELIX IS SMILING AS HE COMES INTO THE room and takes his seat.

'How are you?' he asks me.

'I'm good, thank you Felix.' We sit for a few moments and I notice that I feel pleased to see him and wonder what has happened for him this week.

'I'm leaving.'

'Oh.' I feel a blankness. I didn't expect to hear that today.

'I decided to defer my year. Everyone is very upset.'

'You have deferred for a year and everyone is upset. Who's "everyone"?'

'My tutors, supervisor, my mum.' Felix just stares at the ground for a moment. Then he looks up at me with that grin. 'I had a long chat with my dad at four in the morning after I saw you. I was really upset. He was worried about me and I think he knew how unhappy I was and he said he would help me and support my decision.'

'Wow, Felix, this is huge. How are you feeling?'

'I feel relieved. As Dad said, university isn't going anywhere. He and Mum had a massive row but he said not to worry about that. He said he would help me find a place close to Granny but that I could stay with Granny if I wanted. I think I'm best in my own place close by so I can see her but be independent. I want to try, you know?' I nod. 'It's right, I know it's right.'

'It all feels right for you, Felix.'

'Yeah, and as Dad says, even if it is a romantic dream, what's wrong with that? We need dreams, don't we?'

'We do.'

'It feels so much better knowing that I have his blessing, it really does help me.'

'How does that help you, Felix?'

'It means I'm not on my own.'

'There is someone with you on the dream journey.'

'Exactly that. I didn't realise how alone I felt, which was stupid because I have friends and my tutors have been good but I felt stuck in the black hole.'

'You felt stuck in a black hole, a bit like the black hole you imagined death to be for your granny.'

'*Hoh*, yeah, I forgot about that. Maybe I felt dead somehow and it scared me.'

'It scared you.'

'Like… is this what my life is going to be forever?'

'That was a question you asked yourself?'

'More like a fear I had.'

'And now?'

'I don't feel as scared, which is probably naive I guess, but I feel excited.'

'It's fascinating, isn't it, that the chemical reaction of anxiety is also the same chemical reaction as excitement and somehow we intuitively know the difference between the two states and the meaning for us.'

'Yeah, I never thought about it like that before. I just realised that I don't feel anxious.'

'What do you put that down to, Felix?'

'I guess I'm doing what I want to do and it feels right for me.'

'What might that say about anxiety for you?'

'That it tells me something is wrong or I need something… I dunno, it's like a messenger.'

I hear myself laugh, 'I like that, yeah, I like that description.' We sit for quite a while in silence and I realise that although we have only been in session twenty minutes, we have come to the end.

'My granny is much better. I spoke to her last night. She's happy I'm coming to Paris.'

I smile and nod. We sit a little longer. Felix looks at the clock, we sit a little longer and Felix looks at the clock again.

'I don't know what else to say.'

'So what would you like to do?'

'Well, I just don't think I have anything left to say. I'm leaving tomorrow.'

'You're leaving tomorrow and don't feel you have anything else to say.'

'No. Thank you for everything.'

'You did the work, Felix.'

'Yeah, but thank you.' I nod with gratitude. We sit a little longer and Felix gestures with his hands, palms skyward as if to say "I got nothin'". I smile in acknowledgement. 'I think I'm done.'

'So what would you like to do?'

He points to the door. 'Can I just go?'

'It's your life, Felix, you can do as you please,' I say, smiling but unmoving in my seat.

He grins and hesitates as he lifts out of the chair. When he is standing fully, I stand with him and walk towards the door. As he reaches the door he shakes my hand. 'Thank you,' he says gently.

'Good luck, Felix,' I reply, open the door and out he goes.

Jack

I'M FEELING APPREHENSIVE ABOUT THE NEXT client on my list as it is Jack, from Jack and Christine.

He comes into the room dressed more casually this time in jeans and shirt. He is taller than I remember and less stocky, less solid. I notice his long fingers that look unsure of themselves and I experience a wince of vulnerability in my body.

'Hello Jack. It's good to see you and I'm surprised to see you, to be honest. You were very cross the last time we met. I know you said on the phone that you would be coming on your own to talk and that you don't know if this is a one-off session.'

'Yep, I was really angry with you. I don't know if this is just a one-off, but I wanted to understand what happened in that session.'

'As I said on the phone, I'm happy for this to be a one-off if that is all you need. Can you say more about your anger?'

'Well, you just seemed to sit there and not say very much.'

'You wanted me to say more.'

'See, there you go again.' He *tuts* and swivels his head.

'There I go again?'

'You bat it straight back to me – like you did in that session with Chrissie.'

'It feels like I bat it back – what am I batting, Jack?'

'Well, you're the expert, you tell me.'

'You feel me to be an expert.'

'Oh… fuck… isn't that what you get paid for.'

'You sound exasperated.' I pause then ask, 'Would it be helpful to you to talk about what you want from therapy?'

'Yes! Now we're getting somewhere.'

'That feels like movement to you.'

'Yeah.'

'Movement is important to you?'

'Yeah, and I thought that's what coming here would be about.'

'You thought coming here would be about movement?'

'Yes, is it?'

'Yes, I think therapy can be about change and movement. Though I have to add that none of us know how the movement will come about, what it will look like and what the consequences will be if something does change and move.'

'But there must be predictors or markers or some theory that you work to.'

'Yes, there is a theory of sorts but it is more an underpinning and ethical attitude than a predictive system. And it is complex because there are many models of therapy. You have read about me on my website, do you have any questions about that which might be helpful for you today?'

'No, not really.'

'OK so maybe I can ask a question?' He nods in agreement. 'I'm curious to know what it was about my website that made you choose to come and see me in particular?'

'Well, you were local... erm... I liked the things on your website about exploring etc and, well, you had a nice smile.'

'You like the idea of exploration, felt I had a nice smile and the location was important.'

'Yeah, I mean, it was probably a bit more than that, but when I came off the computer you were the one that stayed in my mind. When I looked again the next day I just liked what you had to say, that it would be confidential and we could explore our relating patterns and stuff.'

'Exploring relating patterns was important to you.'

'Yes, that's why I was a bit miffed when it all got out of hand – you know – I wanted it to be slower.'

'Sure, I can see that, Jack, and that is why you were cross with me. It wasn't slow and it felt like it got out of hand. And you were expecting more from me.' He just nods and takes a sip of his water; shuffles a bit in his seat and looks at his fingers in his lap as though they are talking to him.

'I was expecting more from you.'

'I can appreciate that, I can. Of course, you expected me to do something; I do understand having that expectation. If we had the session again, what specifically would you have liked me to do?'

'Well, I would've liked you to ask some questions.'

'What kind of questions and what would you hope the questions would do?'

'I wanted you to ask about us, me and Chrissie, both of us, so you could get a picture of us together.'

'And what picture would you have liked me to see?'

'Oh God I dunno… that it's not all a bed of roses and that I've worked hard to keep the family going.'

'Your marriage is not a bed of roses and you have worked hard for the family.'

'Yeah, I work pretty long hours, you know. And I know Chrissie has been with the kids and everything but sometimes… sometimes I don't think she really sees the stress I've been under and the energy it takes to keep everything going.'

'You'd like Chrissie to see how stressful life is for you sometimes and how much it takes to keep everything going. If she could see that, and I could've done something that would've brought that about in that first session, what would be different now do you think?'

'We, we'd both be sat here working it through.'

'You would both be here working it through.'

'Yes, our marriage,' he tears up, 'I love Chrissie, I do, I can't imagine life without her, it makes no sense to me.'

'It makes no sense to you, the thought of life without Chrissie, and yet you engage in a number of affairs that risk having to live life without her.'

'I know, I know. I just. You know. I'm attracted to other women and it takes some of the stress off and… I dunno, I feel freer somehow.'

'Freer.'

'From the hassles and pressure of keeping everything going… it's not just that… I like the women, I care for them, I do. I didn't know that Chrissie knew as much she did. I was a bit taken aback actually.'

'You care for the women and were taken aback that Chrissie knew so much.'

'Mmm… I think that's another reason why I was angry with you. It was like you revealed me… I know you didn't but that's what it felt like. And I couldn't get angry with Chrissie, though she blew everything out of context.'

'What do you mean out of context?'

'Well she just launched in all guns blazing, I just…'

'You just?'

'She caught me off guard. I had prepared how I was going to say things and I felt bashed… you know, really put on the spot.'

'It all went too fast, you were bashed and caught off-guard and couldn't say what you had intended to say. I'm hearing something about you had your speech prepared.'

He laughs with a half-hearted grin. 'It wasn't like a speech. I just had an idea in my mind that you'd ask questions and I knew what I was going to say and we would gradually get into looking at our marriage. Instead… well, you know…' We sit in silence for a moment or two whilst he looks down at his fingers. He lifts his head and looks at me, still rolling his fingers. 'I'm sorry I was so mad with you, especially when I threw the money down.' He drops his head slightly.

'I'm curious about your apology.'

'I wasn't mad with you really, was I?'

'You don't feel that you were mad with me.'

'No, I was mad with... I... dunno... me I suppose. I was so... on the back foot... misjudged everything... Chrissie overpowered me with what she knew. You know, I sit in some pretty aggressive board meetings and don't get thrown like that.'

'You felt overpowered by Chrissie and were mad with yourself.'

'I felt, oh I dunno, she shocked me.'

'You felt shocked.'

'I did, yeah. And a bit ashamed that she had known all this time.'

'You felt ashamed.' He sits looking down at his hands.

'I guess I took advantage not realising she knew all along anyway, so when she said what she said.' He puffs through his cheeks, forcing a gust of air out through his mouth, head bowed. 'Reminded me of my mum.'

'Something reminded you of your mum.'

'Yeah, my dad was a cheater too and when we were all grown up, she just left... walked out... said enough.'

'How old were you when she left?'

'I was sixteen, Alan, my brother, was eighteen. It was like *fuck* – where did that come from, you know – no warning, just gone.' He goes quite red in the face.

'That was a shock too, no warning, gone, similar to Chrissie's response – no warning and her revelation was out.'

Jack sits for a few moments. He takes a sip of water. Looking at his hands he lets his head fall back against the seat, and in a quiet voice says, 'In that session, I felt the same age, felt sixteen all over again. I couldn't catch my thoughts and didn't really know what to say. Which is why I kept looking at you, hoping you would do something. I guess I just reacted.'

'You just reacted, felt young and lost your words. It was a powerful moment, I remember your struggle. I'm sorry that I didn't do more that might have helped both of you at that moment.' He stares at me and I'm not sure what that last statement means to him, but his stare has taken him somewhere. He continues to stare at me and then smiles.

'I just realised. You look a bit like her.'

'Like who?'

'My mum.'

'I look like your mum?'

'Yeah, not really, something, I dunno, reminds me.'

'What's it like for you to sit with someone who reminds you of your mum?'

'A bit mixed. I mean we have a good relationship, I think. Sometimes I think I'm still angry that she left. I met Chrissie soon after and we got married and had the kids, and... I don't know, life just seemed to happen.'

'You speak as though you had no agency, no choices, and that things happened quickly.'

'They did. Don't get me wrong, I loved Chrissie, still do, but... my mum... you know...'

'Finish the sentence Jack, your mum...' He looks into the air, around the room, at his fingers trying to find the words or else mediate the ones he has in his mind.

'She left. It was hard. I don't think anybody realised how hard it was.' He cries a little and I sit with him amidst the tears sneaking away down his red face.

'It was hard for you and it felt like nobody noticed. Sounds lonely.'

Jack blows his nose and straightens himself up in the seat.

'She's seeing someone,' he whispers.

'Who's seeing someone?'

'Chrissie.'

'I notice I feel a little surprised. It wasn't something I expected to hear today.'

'Been going on a long time apparently. I'm not surprised. She had a fling just before we got married. I found out the day before the wedding, nearly didn't go through with it, but you know, you do. I think there have been others. That's why that day when we were here I wanted to look at it all, slowly 'cause I knew she'd put on that front. But...' I wait for him to finish that thought. 'But she would never look at anything. She created this image of the perfect wife and family but it was bollocks, just bollocks, and she beat me for it.'

'You felt beaten.'

'Yeah, battered. Battered. She'd scream sometimes, hysterical even, with such venom, not often but it would come out of nowhere. No one else knew, as far as the world's concerned we have a perfect marriage'

'To the world your marriage is perfect yet in reality you feel battered.' He glares a momentary stillness, looks at his shoes and shuffles in his seat.

'Yeah, I mean it was OK… sometimes in between the screaming, you know, but yeah that's the impression we gave everyone I guess. You do, don't you – pretend?'

'You pretended to the world, and maybe to each other?'

'To be honest, I never really knew where I was, what I was gonna face when I got in.'

'Sounds precarious, like walking on eggshells.'

'Yeah it was, but I just went with it and tried to make things calm, you know, for the kids as well.'

'Your role was to calm things.'

'Yeah… didn't always work.' He grins and eyes become teary at the same time.

'What happened when it didn't work?'

'She'd throw something or have a full-on tantrum, she hits out at me sometimes and sometimes she'd just leave the house and go out on a bit of a bender with friends.'

'What was that like for you?'

'I just got on with it, I'd look after the kids.'

'You took care of things.'

'Somebody had to. I think it really affects the kids.'

'And you, how does it affect you?'

'To be honest, I'd be kinda relieved. Me and the kids would settle down eventually, order a takeaway and watch a movie. We're close.'

'There was relief when Chrissie left the house. You and the children could settle.'

'Don't get me wrong, Chrissie could be lovely too. I just, just wanted us to get to the bottom of all this so we could have more of the good stuff.'

'You feel if you could go deep enough, you could get to the bottom of the issue and have more of the good stuff in your marriage.'

'Isn't that the point of therapy?'

'I don't always buy into the idea that there is a bottom to get to and, once revealed, all will be well. I think we have to deal with the here and now and acknowledge our experiencing in the moment when we encounter another person.'

'So, I really need Chrissie to be here in other words.'

'Well, it would be an advantage to be able to work with you both as you each experience the rise and fall of your relationship in the moment. But, equally, you and I can work together to get more of an understanding of what motivates you and triggers you to respond in certain ways. At least that way you can be more in touch with your own feelings and desires when relating to Chrissie.'

'Sounds complex.'

'Well I guess in one way it is, and yet, in another it's really simple, because if you can connect with your experience in the moment, you can give yourself even just a nanosecond to choose how to respond rather than just reacting to one another.'

I notice his stillness and make him aware that the session has almost run out of time. He states that he wants his marriage to survive and wants to come back to therapy with Chrissie if she will agree, and that if she doesn't, then he'd like to carry on working with me on his own. He remains in his seat when he pays me at the end of the session.

As I ready the room for my next client, I think about Tess, as a letter had arrived this morning enclosing a card from her. The letter was from her daughter informing me that Tess had "passed away peacefully in the hospice" on August 30th. Tess had written a card for me to say thank you for "our conversation" that day back in June. She had written that she'd felt "something has both left my body and entered all at the same time… that something was love." She stated that she'd felt lucky to have had the life she did, that she regretted nothing and feels ready to meet Ted, her deceased husband, whom she knew would be waiting at the lift. She joked and wrote, "I hope the joke's not on us and it's a concrete box after all!"

Afterword

ALL LIFE IS A WITHSTANDING; A PANTOMIME THAT we experience at the very core of our belly and outer layer of our skin. We unavoidably encounter the world at every moment, not as observers from a velvet seat in the dress circle, but as embodied conscious beings on a stage already constructed. Therapy can be a way in; an open invitation to explore our moment-to-moment unyielding and compulsory movement through each act of this thing called life.

Like us, therapy itself is an accident waiting to happen. As therapists, we have no way of knowing what a therapeutic shift for any client will be, and mostly we are not privy to the moment of shift, we only get to hear the reporting of it. These significant moments leave an imprint on and within a person. An accidental, yet indelible marking. In a way, this is symbolic of the accidental nature of existence itself: the conception, the birthing, the growth, every twist and turn. We are not fixed things but experiments in constant movement. Whilst in therapy we may find words and descriptions that match our experience, they may also change over time and so we are in a constant state of editing our narrative, our lived experience and the meaning we make of it in any given moment. The impermanence of our moment-to-moment living reveals the absurdity and decay of our existence. But oh what joy, to wake to the wind and rain, the sun and warmth; to bask in the wonder of all encounter, and the accident that is all existence.

Hospitality

In the end, it is simple:
Love and be loved.
Our journey to figure out
how. Experience between the
sheets; caring in sickness;
supporting the stranger within,
and without; knowing
the distance between us is no
distance at all; that moment of
remembrance as we gasp our last?
Love…
begins with H.

Acknowledgements

NOTHING THAT IS WRITTEN HERE IS REAL; ALL IS fiction, the reality of which is visceral, and these ideas are derived from those teachers, artists, poets, writers and musicians who have inspired me. The most impactful include:

Manu Bazzano, Judith Butler, Ludwig Wittgenstein, Friedrich Nietzsche, Jean-Paul Sartre, Simone de Beauvoir, Gilles Deleuze, Brian Massumi, Carl Rogers, David Bowie, Leonard Cohen, Bob Dylan, Joni Mitchell, Guy Garvey, Jorie Graham, Philip Roth, Hanif Kureishi, Mary Wesley, Shunyru Suzuki, Taizan Maezumi, Thich Nhat Hanh, and many practitioners and writers of Zen Buddhism.

I thank chance that their work was on the path that I have walked so far and thank them for bothering to make their mark that my eyes and ears became alert to.

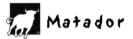 Matador

For exclusive discounts on Matador titles,
sign up to our occasional newsletter at
troubador.co.uk/bookshop